Praise for *Your Mental*

'I worked with Zoë for six mont[...] always been quite sceptical about wheue[...] from therapy. During that time, she helped me to get to know myself, understand myself and be kinder to myself.'
– Dr Zoë Williams

'Zoë's techniques are easy and give great results. Her work has given me wonderful insight into how I can look after my mind and makes mental wellness feel accessible to everyone. I highly recommend *Your Mental Health Workout* to anyone who has the desire to improve their emotional health.'
– Pixie Lott

'This is a well-developed pattern, a sure-fire plan and a riveting must-read if success in your chosen field is important to you.'
– Derrick Evans AKA Mr Motivator

'*Your Mental Health Workout* has had a massive positive impact on our clients.'
– Tatum Getty, Marketing Director of Barry's Bootcamp

'*Your Mental Health Workout* is an invaluable, easily digestible and accessible guide to maintaining mental health.'
– Founder and Director of GroOops Dyslexia Aware Counselling

'She makes therapy easy to understand, access and benefit from. Her focus on specific and measurable workouts means anyone who wants to, can get the results they are after.'
– Aimie Atkinson

YOUR
MENTAL
HEALTH
Workout

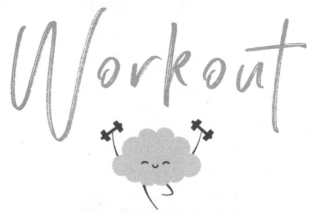

A 5 Week Programme to a
Healthier, Happier Mind

ZOË ASTON

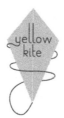

Your Mental Health Workout is suitable for everyone, at any stage of life and at any stage in their health journey. It is not, however, a replacement for treatment, therapy or medication, nor can it promise to heal you or change your life – just to make you feel happier and healthier within it. This is just one stop on your mental health journey.

If you are experiencing thoughts of harming yourself or others or suspect that you need further professional help, please take the initiative to seek it beyond this book. You can find a list of resources for additional support on p. 231.

First published in Great Britain in 2021 by Yellow Kite
An Imprint of Hodder & Stoughton
An Hachette UK company

3

A CIP catalogue record for this title is available from the British Library

Trade Paperback ISBN 978 1 529 35406 5
eBook ISBN 978 1 529 35405 8

Typeset in Celeste by Palimpsest Book Production Ltd, Falkirk, Stirlingshire

Printed and bound in Great Britain by Clays Ltd, Elcograf S.p.A.

Hodder & Stoughton policy is to use papers that are natural, renewable and recyclable products and made from wood grown in sustainable forests. The logging and manufacturing processes are expected to conform to the environmental regulations of the country of origin.

Yellow Kite
Hodder & Stoughton Ltd
Carmelite House
50 Victoria Embankment
London EC4Y 0DZ

www.yellowkitebooks.co.uk

CONTENTS

INTRODUCTION

WELCOME TO YOUR Mental Health Workout: A 5-Week Programme to a Healthier, Happier Mind.

Historically, in order to get help with their mental health, a person would have been referred for therapy, taking place with a therapist, in a dedicated room, behind closed doors. As a result, therapy became stigmatised as something that we only do when we are unwell or there is a specific problem. The notion that we only work on our mental health at these times gives us the message, when we do look for help, that there is something wrong *with us*! And it is this messaging that has caused us to feel shame around asking for support – shame around the possibility that there is something going on with our minds that we are unable to cope with; and shame around not being 'good enough'. This is what drives exactly the parts of us that need attention further into hiding.

If there was something 'wrong' with your body – if you had a headache, a broken wrist, a tummy ache or something even more sinister – you'd most likely either know how to treat it or seek out the relevant help without too much difficulty. Mental health should be the same. I want all of us to know exactly what to do when we feel sad, anxious or depressed and when we are grieving or there is a big change happening. I want to supply the kit and skills needed to cope with difficult life transitions, to understand and adjust unhelpful or self-destructive behaviours. I want to make your mind a happier place to be.

Because of the stigma that to some extent still surrounds getting psychological help, many people try to use willpower in an attempt to control the things they are ashamed of (and have no reason to be) and prove that they are 'strong' enough to 'beat' it. But if you use willpower and brute force in an attempt to 'fix' your mind, it will, like any other muscle, fatigue and collapse quickly, causing you to resort to old, unhelpful, unhappy behaviours.

Your Mental Health Workout will help you to develop consistency, commitment, accountability and responsibility for your psychological wellbeing, so you do not have to rely on willpower alone. It supports you in seeking and navigating both internal and external maintenance systems, leaving you feeling more energised, with better knowledge about your own mental health and armed with the tools you need to feel happier and healthier in the long run.

My mission is to help change the way we approach mental health, taking therapy outside of the therapy room and making psychological work available wherever you are. Having the tools to work on your mental health is not a privilege – it's a human right.

Having said all this, over the past decade there has been a huge increase in the number of people talking about mental health. There have also been many significant changes to the way we function as a society which have challenged us and opened our minds. We have seen people of all ages speak out about their mental health struggles and boldly share how they cope and what help they receive, if any. The millennials, in particular, and those who have followed, have helped to change things. They are eager to heal and tell people about it, busting the stigma and shame that have been attached to mental health, talking about difficult things and laying the groundwork for less stigma going forward. It is my belief that the millennial generation, and Gen Z in particular, are attempting to heal from not only the destructive effects of challenging events in their own lifetimes, but also the traumas of the generations before them that have been left unaddressed, negatively impacting mental health in the present day.

There is also a new breed of therapist on the rise – the millennial therapist – of which I am one. We want to make an impact, and with our familiarity with social media we can reach people across the globe. Mental health bloggers, vloggers, advocates and campaigners have also made a massive difference to how we support each other psychologically. But there are, relatively speaking, just a handful with the qualifications and extensive experience required to provide accessible information and treatment to all who need it. This is important, as there are thousands of people on social media offering advice, but many are not qualified to do so.

This is where Your Mental Health Workout comes in: a 5-week plan that promises to move you towards a happier, healthier and calmer mind. And it works – for anyone who is motivated enough to stay committed and trust the process.

Just like any other personal development journey, if motivation and commitment are exactly the things you struggle with, we will work on them too.

This all started when I became aware of all the information available about what to eat and how to eat it, what type of exercise to do in order to get specific results and how readily all this information is consumed. There is a lot of information about mental health out there too, but nothing that really tells you exactly what to do, how to do it and what to expect. How come we have so much information about looking after our bodies and not our minds? Your Mental Health Workout is uniquely structured to fill this gap. It is an easy and actionable programme – something I wish I had had put in front of me all those years ago when I was struggling with my own mental health.

Of course, there are nuances for each individual and I hope this programme allows for that. Generally the steps here are directive and specific and also designed with the awareness that you need the space to find ways to make this work for *your* mind.

Psychological wellbeing should be available to everyone, regardless of age, gender, sexuality, economic status, race or religion. I shudder when I hear about people with eating disorders who cannot get funded treatment because they are not considered 'sick enough' and when I see those with other psychiatric issues not receiving the robust support they need. And I also feel disappointed that so many of those who just want to take better care of their mental health don't have access to or even know how to use the available support systems. I want that to change. That's why this programme is designed for anyone and everyone – those who want to achieve an overall enhanced sense of mental wellbeing, as well as those who want to target specific problems.

About Me

Born in London in 1987, I am the eldest of two, my sister being five years younger than me. I lived with my sister and parents until I was twenty, when my mental health was at its worst and we all agreed I could no longer live at home.

What happened during those twenty years is a challenge to put down on paper, but I'd like to fill you in a bit, so you know where I am coming from.

I was a painfully shy child, who could hardly speak. I still remember that shyness now; it is visceral. I attached myself to the ankles of my mother for the best part of the first ten years of my life and have always struggled with attachment and separation anxiety. Through the years, I sought out intense attachments in teachers, mentors and friends. I was searching for something to make me feel loved and whole from a very early stage in my development.

School was tough. I just couldn't keep up academically and was diagnosed with dyslexia when I was eight years old. I was lucky that this was identified early, and I received the assistance and support I required to get through the basic academia during primary and secondary school.

School is not something I look back on fondly. I moved around a lot – partly because of the dyslexia and trying to find somewhere that could help me learn in a way that made sense to me, and partly because when I was thirteen, I was on the receiving end of some pretty horrendous bullying. This left a mental health scar I am not sure will ever fully heal.

Although I believe I always struggled with my mental health – that it is, in part, to do with genetics and does, indeed, run in my family – it was the mixture of difficulties at home, academic challenges, painful attachments with friends and this experience of being bullied colliding that resulted in the symptoms of my mental health decline. In order to survive, my only option was to shut down on myself. I became depressed and anxious and I lost faith in those who were supposed to protect me.

Sooner rather than later (thankfully), I left the school I was bullied at and went to a stage school, which is what I had always wanted. I wanted to dance! But a year on, I started self-harming and making myself vomit. I was fourteen.

Between the ages of fourteen and twenty I was diagnosed with a number of things, including – but not limited to – eating disorders (in as many forms as you can imagine – undereating, overeating, purging in a variety of ways) and self-harm. Both these behaviours helped me to manage the anxiety and depression that I was living with, but eventually they became my main troubles as I lost control of my behaviour. Throughout various stints in therapy and rehab I was told I was addicted, had a personality disorder, lacked a conscience.

I am not big on labels these days. They can be very helpful, but ultimately, it was only when I understood that my mental health was as much a part of me as my body and that I had to find the skills to support it in a way that was sustainable for me, that I got better.

Things were very up and down in those adolescent years. I had a turbulent relationship with my family while suffering from my eating disorder, and because I was so desperately insecure and either behaving compulsively or isolating myself in order to cope with being alive, I did not make or hold on to many friends. Despite all of this, I was relatively successful in setting up a dance company when I was sixteen. In many ways, I used dance and choreography to express my inner world because I had found no other way of doing it. I really wish people had been talking about mental health back then as openly as we are now. There was so much shame for both me and my family about what was going on and that just exacerbated the issue.

I struggled to make friendships throughout this time because my compulsive behaviours and the way they helped me cope were far more important to me than connecting with others; maybe this is why I am so eager now to help people understand the importance of connection – both with ourselves and others. I also feel that the level of separation anxiety I experienced and the mental scars from the bullying, among other traumas, left me unable to imagine why people would want to be friends with me. I hated myself so much . . . how could anyone else possibly like me?

Because of this I have very few friends who have seen me on both sides of my mental health journey. I had to build up my support network as an adult and my family and I often talk about how extraordinary it is that I am, basically, a totally different person now. It is the internal work that made a huge difference to how I treat myself. That painfully shy child, the teenager full of shame and self-loathing – they are still in there; but I have learned to care for them internally, so that I can fulfil my potential in my external world. It may sound cheesy, but it's true: as long as I take good care of myself, my potential appears to be endless. Sometimes I wonder if it was this that frightened me about being alive.

The people who were there for all of this were, of course, my family. We are a pretty solid unit of four, but boy, have we had a rough ride in terms of mental health, and family dynamics are difficult. Each of us has our own stuff, and we have all contributed to each other's highs and lows. It was my family who bore the brunt of living with someone who had an eating disorder and was self-harming, and it was they who witnessed my decline.

Just after I turned twenty, we agreed I needed more help. I had already been in therapy on and off throughout my life, and regularly since I was eighteen. We decided I would go to an in-patient treatment programme for my eating disorder. I thought I was going for a week . . . I stayed for a year.

While in treatment, doing intensive therapy each day, I learned more about myself than most do in a lifetime. I worked on my relationships with my body, my mind, my history, my relationships with others, my attachments. I was young enough that I had the time to invest in my recovery – I can't say it was a pleasant experience, but the results in the years to follow were definitely worth the challenge.

Coming back into my life was not easy either; I struggled for many years afterwards. What that intensive experience gave me were the foundations to build my life on. I continued with my dancing for a couple of years. Then, one day, I found myself sitting in a park realising that my mind was not made for the dance industry. My mental health was not improving, and I couldn't see it working for me in the long run. On a whim, I decided to apply to university to get a master's degree in psychology and counselling.

I was turned away the first time I applied because, at twenty-two, they said I was too young for the master's course and lacking in life experience. It was suggested that I do a foundation year in psychology or counselling to see if I enjoyed the subject and wanted to commit to four years of studying. Throughout 2009, I followed that advice, while continuing with my dancing career. I went back the next year, still committed to the subject, and they gave me a place. I knew I'd found my calling when the same night that I was worrying about funding the course I got a call to say I had been successful in one of the scholarship applications I'd submitted, The Esmond Robinson Scholarship. I am forever grateful and still have a strong relationship with the couple who funded my master's.

I finished my master's degree in psychology in 2013, when I was twenty-six, and I was lucky enough to find work in treatment centres as a group and one-to-one therapist, working with eating disorders, addictions and trauma. I loved it. It was tough and draining, and I cried most days for the first few years, but it was both invaluable experience and very rewarding at the same time. It is this work and all the people I have met along the way – other mental health professionals and clients alike – that have contributed to not only my professional skill set but my own mental wellbeing too.

Nowadays, I work independently in private practice and I consult for brands, companies and teams in the UK to help bring mental health to the forefront.

How to Use This Book

The unique blend of my own mental health struggles and my work as a therapist and mental health consultant is what qualifies me to create and promote the ideas that underpin Your Mental Health Workout. In the programme, I draw together the effective parts of therapeutic healing and use the workout metaphor to explain complex psychological concepts in a way that everyone can understand.

If you read my eBook during the 2020 pandemic, *Your Mental Health First Aid Kit: Quick and Easy Techniques for Coming Out of Lockdown*, you'll already have a vague idea about what is going to happen here. Like any good training programme, it is important you know what the plan looks like and how to use it; it is even more important that you identify the results you want to get out of it – for you.

You might be tempted to flick through the book and jump to the workouts you like the sound of. If that is the case, consider the following questions:

- What is a feeling?
- What exactly is a thought?
- Do you feel in control of your behaviours?
- How do you create and maintain self-esteem?

If you are unsure of any of the answers, you'll need to read the book from start to finish. In fact, regardless of whether you *think* you know the answers right now or not, I'd suggest you read the book in its entirety.

After laying the groundwork, which will help you to under-stand what mental health actually means, without judgment or stigma or specific diagnoses attached to it, we will set your mental health goals, followed by a warm-up and then eight different mental health workouts. I will introduce you to each one in detail and explain *how* and *why* we are doing them.

All the workouts included here involve techniques that I have learned over my time as a therapist and as a human being on the same planet as you. I have mixed together various therapeutic models and concepts from pioneers in the wellness industry, as well as my own mentors', and pack-aged them in an easy-to-understand metaphor. Each 'workout' is designed to build on the last, and although each can be used in isolation, you will experience a happier and healthier mind if you follow the structure offered to you here. Put simply: work on your mind in the same way that you would your body.

Every chapter leads with the workout steps, followed by the 'why' we do it and the 'how' to get it working for you. You'll also notice I ask questions about you throughout. The intention behind this is to keep your focus on you. All too often, when we gather new information, we immediately start assigning it to other people in our lives: 'Oh, my mum has that', 'My brother would benefit from this', 'That's what was up with my friend that time' . . . I want your focus here to be on you.

One way to enhance your experience of this programme is to do it alongside another person or even a group of people. You can use each other as workout partners to ensure your focus stays where you need it to be, and it also helps to make you accountable to someone other than yourself. Of course, this is optional, and the programme will work just as well if you prefer to do it as an individual.

The last practical part of the book contains two appendices, comprising a physio section for your feelings, along with some modifications and progressions for some specific mental health ailments. This is where you can dip in and out to get what you need when you need it. If you do notice a particular bias towards a feeling, judgment or disposition, making it difficult to see opportunities for change, this section can support you with moving through this; use it to help strengthen those parts of your mind that seem to be having more trouble than others.

Along the way are some myth busters, where we break down some of the stigma around mental health and take the time to understand the reality of what goes on in our minds and why we no longer need to feel afraid of it. These are designed as stand-alone pages, but will also be relevant to the workouts in which they appear. And every now and again during this process I offer you journaling opportunities, too.

Finally, should anything in particular have sparked your interest, you will find a comprehensive section at the back of this book to inspire any further reading, as well as a list of resources for additional support.

Despite the aim here being for you to eventually include all eight mental health workouts over a period of five weeks, I would first encourage you to take things slowly, introducing each workout as and when you feel ready. There's nothing more demotivating than being overwhelmed by a new process. I encourage self-respect, gentleness and kindness throughout. If your mental health is something you have never paid this much attention to, start small and do what you can, just as you would with any other muscle. Your full five weeks might come a little further down the line than it does for others, and I completely and kindly support you in that. Please carry this kindness with you; it is the most underrated but powerful agent of human change.

After you've completed your first full five weeks, you can decide what works for you: what you'd like to integrate into your life going forward and what you'd rather leave behind.

USING THE CHECKLIST AND PLANNERS

You will find planners and a checklist on pp. xxi–xxvi. These are also available to download via my website (see p. 233). You are welcome to print them off as many times as you like and use them as you see fit. There are also checklists at the end of each workout. These are in no way intended to point out whether you are doing it 'wrong' or 'right'; they are simply suggestions, and you may find a different way that works best for you.

In fact, there is no wrong or right, although you can make it tougher on yourself (and not in a helpful way) if you are not honest about how you approach the programme, the level you work at and the effort you hold yourself accountable to. One of the major ways we create dishonesty for ourselves in this sense, is when we make these changes for someone other than ourselves. You must be working on your mental health for the good of *yourself.* Your Mental Health Workout is YOURS! It will not save your relationship, change your mother or make your friends behave differently. It is true that people around you may benefit from the positive changes you make, but that has to be a bonus effect of you working on yourself for yourself.

The trick is to be curious about what makes a particular workout easier or more challenging for you. You can use the planners to identify any patterns, habits and cycles. The more interested you are in yourself along the way, the more you will learn and the more opportunities for change you will create.

Just like a physical workout, if you get tired, lose momentum or your commitment falters, you can pick up where you left off at any time – no judgment involved. Just start a new planner and remember that maximum change happens when you are focused, committed and challenged. There's a phrase in fitness: 'fight fatigue with focus' – and that is all the planners and checklists are there to do: to keep you focused. When you get tired, focus in on something specific. For example, if your energy levels are such that all you can do for a few days are a couple of gratitudes or a minute's worth of mindfulness each day, then do those and really stick to them, while the rest of you recovers.

Mental health doesn't really take time out, but rest days are totally part of the plan!

The checklist opposite allows you to tick off each workout as and when you have completed it. You can update it each week.

The five weekly planners overleaf will help you to schedule and structure Your Mental Health Workout around your life.

YOUR MENTAL HEALTH WORKOUT WEEKLY CHECKLIST

WEEKLY WORKOUTS	M	T	W	TH	F	S	SU
THERAPY							
SOCIAL EVENTS							
EXERCISE							
SELF-CARE							

DAILY WORKOUTS							
MINDFULNESS							
CONNECTION							
APPRECIATION							
MOVEMENT							

WEEK 1 PLANNER

Use this page to plan when your workouts will take place

MON	TUE	WED	THU	FRI	SAT	SUN

What changes have you noticed this week?

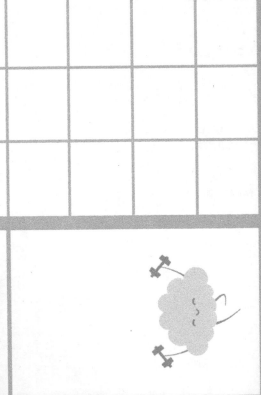

WEEK 2 PLANNER

Use this page to plan when your workouts will take place

MON	TUE	WED	THU	FRI	SAT	SUN

What changes have you noticed this week?

WEEK 3 PLANNER

Use this page to plan when your workouts will take place

MON	TUE	WED	THU	FRI	SAT	SUN

What changes have you noticed this week?

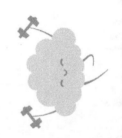

WEEK 4 PLANNER

Use this page to plan when your workouts will take place

MON	TUE	WED	THU	FRI	SAT	SUN

What changes have you noticed this week?

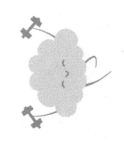

WEEK 5 PLANNER

Use this page to plan when your workouts will take place

	MON	TUE	WED	THU	FRI	SAT	SUN

What changes have you noticed this week?

Use these, or print copies off from my website and stick them somewhere visible to you – say, on your fridge or by your bedside. Or you can even take a picture of them on your phone and put them in your favourites, so you can fill them in and access them with ease.

Working on your mental health is not all flowers and rainbows. It is pretty hard work some of the time and, thankfully, there is an online community of people who can support you at www.instagram.com/yourmentalhealthworkout. Please do share your journey with us.

You, and everyone else around you, right now, deserve the opportunity to focus on having a healthy mind. Together, we can open up new possibilities to help us allow and acknowledge our own feelings and thoughts about life, make healthy emotional connections and experience the present moment as it is, right now, rather than colouring it with historic experiences. And by changing the unhelpful beliefs, attitudes and behaviours we cling to, we can see the world in a whole new way. This book is where we begin.

MENTAL HEALTH MYTH

*'You can overcome difficulty using willpower
and discipline alone'*

It is true that willpower is a good starting point for most changes you want to make in life. Nevertheless, changes in your mental health, good and bad, are not something that always happen consciously or have anything to do with the essence of who you are. That is, your mental health difficulties do not define you or tell us anything about your worth or willpower.

In part, busting the stigma around mental health also means helping people to understand that when thoughts, feelings and behaviours are in question, if we can 'snap out of it' using willpower we will tend to do that. Yet most often, we actually can't. It's not as simple as stopping 'if you try hard enough' with mental health stuff – because a lot of it is less conscious than we appreciate. You wouldn't be able to recover from a physical wound just by telling it to stop being injured. The same goes for psychological healing. We are not always in control of our minds and we do not always have a say in how long they take to heal. The workouts in this book will get you to a place where you have more choice over your mental health; they will create windows of opportunity for healing that bypass the issue of how much willpower or self-discipline you have.

PART ONE

UNDERSTANDING MENTAL HEALTH

Chapter 1: Getting to Know Your Mental Health

Chapter 2: Goal Setting

Chapter 1

GETTING TO KNOW
YOUR MENTAL HEALTH

THE MIND NEEDS as much of a workout as the body, and I have found that when judgment and jargon are removed and we destigmatise mental health, people feel empowered to take more care of their minds and allow themselves to create goals, so that they can work towards achieving the results they desire. It is not an easy road to take, I'll give you that. Anyone who invests time and energy in their mental health knows how active you need to be around it, and has my utmost respect.

Throughout this programme the metaphor of the mind as a muscle is used to draw a comparison with physical workout programmes to help you understand simple ways of moving towards a happier, healthier mind. It is important to note, however, that the brain, in reality, is an organ, and is far more complex than any muscle in the body. It is what contains your mind and what we refer to as your mental health.

With regards to the body–mind comparison, Your Mental Health Workout will help you to consider them as one entity.

3

We tend to think of the mind as being separate from the body, but it is part of it. I would love for people to add the mind into their physical training programmes as a matter of course: arm day, leg day, full-body day, rest day and brain day!

Most of us have tried changing our bodies at one time or another because we believe it will make us happier and healthier. (And it might.) But if our minds are out of shape, it is unlikely that we will be able to see our bodies for what they are and feel content with them. Changes in the physical body are hugely dependent on mindset, so while the focus on body works in the short term, we can sometimes treat them as a short cut to 'health', and they become the target for the unprocessed things going on in our minds. This leads to mental health declines, as evidenced by the rise of eating disorders of all kinds, increased reports of anxiety and more and more people coming forward with stress-related physical troubles like irritable bowel syndrome, panic attacks, hair loss, insomnia, muscle soreness and skin problems. I cannot tell you how many clients I have seen who have already consulted every other type of health practitioner, taken every type of vitamin, adjusted their nutrition and had more than their fair share of attempts at fixing what's going on in their minds via external forces, such as changing jobs, taking time out, moving house, ending relationships, starting relationships – the list goes on. Then they come to therapy and discover that they are carrying heavy emotional loads that need processing. The way we look after our minds and our internal world clearly needs to be addressed alongside how

4

we look after our bodies and use external factors to keep us happy.

Working on your mental health is about being curious and open to learning about how your mind works. At times, clients have come to me for therapy and we have both been surprised at how quickly they heal. One client, years ago, arrived with a huge weight on their shoulders, feeling so unable to take any more that they felt they were only staying alive for those who relied on them. It was desperately sad. Yet all they needed to hear was that they were allowed to prioritise themselves – to put themselves first. No one had ever suggested this to them. All of a sudden, their self-esteem seemed to kick in, boundaries were easier to hold and their emotional wellbeing was on the mend. They already had the answers inside of them, but just needed help accessing them.

Of course, there are other situations where it has taken far longer to figure out what works, what heals and what hinders. Your Mental Health Workout is effective at both ends of this scale and everywhere in between. It is the exploration of your mind that allows us to understand what works best for you. But how do we do this?

Rather than go into the neuroscience here, I want to break down mental health within the context of our workout metaphor, keeping our attention on the things we can all easily observe, have experienced and can connect on, namely:

- thoughts
- feelings
- behaviour.

Thoughts

Thoughts are the words that we think, the way we speak to ourselves and others. They are how we communicate ideas and tell people about ourselves and about decisions we've made. Our thinking is generally under our conscious control and is a great place for us to start because it sits exactly in between our feelings and behaviours, both of which we will cover next. You have more control over your thinking than you do feelings and behaviours, so learning how to notice, challenge and change it without judgment is, if nothing else, a handy lifestyle skill and fundamental to living a mindful life. To do this, you must be open to changing your thinking if it appears that something different would be more supportive for you. Sounds easy, but it's complicated for a number of reasons . . .

The way we think is affected by our history. For example, if you grew up with a family or peers who thought mental health was important, you are likely to think in a similar way; likewise, if you grew up in a family who did not think mental health was important you will also think in a similar way. The way we think allows us to connect with our families and peer groups throughout our development. Therefore, changing it is multifaceted because not only are you admitting that what is so familiar is not working for you, but you are also letting go of notions you have believed about how you 'fit in'. The good news is that as you start to notice your thinking and where it comes from, you begin to hold yourself accountable for the changes you want to make, taking responsibility for the thinking part of your mind. This is a process of change, separation and growing into the person you want to be; you are letting go of thought patterns that no longer align with you.

You probably already know that most of our verbal communication with each other involves turning thoughts into words that allow us to portray our emotional landscape: angry, sad, happy, excited, etc. You'll also know a lot of words to explain things that are happening in your physical body: headache, tummy ache, well rested, tired, hungry, hurt, etc. This way of communicating is vital to the survival of human beings, as it means, from a very early stage in our development, we can convey our thoughts and collectively solve problems. However, thoughts can also cause us some trouble, particularly when they are affected by a difficult history and when they evolve into cognitive distortions, which, during this programme, will be known as 'cognitive pulls', negative self-talk and unhelpful judgments.

It is useful to know that our thoughts are not always facts. When I am working with people in therapy, it doesn't actually matter so much if what they think or how they remember something is accurate and factual; what matters is how it affects their thinking – what they do with the reality they are experiencing and how they communicate it.

Thoughts are Your Mental Health Workout equipment. They are to be used with caution and understood fully. When you understand how to use this equipment, you can navigate it in an effective way, without risk of injury, and learn how to challenge and change it. With this knowledge and understanding, you are then able to honestly

7

communicate what you need from others and explain how they can be helpful and supportive of you (no one's mental health equipment works in exactly the same way as the next person's). You will get a better handle on this when we warm up your psychological range of motion on p. 32. Modifications in how you use your equipment are an excellent way to spot changes in your mental health. Throughout the next five weeks, I will explain, and we will discover how your equipment can be used to support your mental health and create a strong and steady mind. We will look at any thoughts that have been pulled in painful and unhelpful directions and how they limit you. You will be supported to move past the thinking blocks and limitations you set for yourself and find a way of thinking about things that is realistic and helpful.

There are as many different ways of thinking as there are people on the planet. A common frustration that comes up for all of us is that we sometimes find it difficult to understand that other people do not think in the same way as we do. This can be the cause of miscommunication and crossed lines in relationships. Which is why, when you do therapy, your therapist helps you to focus on and learn about your own thinking patterns, so that you know what to look out for: the good, the bad and the ugly. When you have a handle on your own thinking, it is far easier to be around other people without the expectation that they, by default, know what is going on in your mind.

In order to better understand your thinking patterns, it is helpful to conceptualise them through three different weight categories: short-lived, long-lived and intrusive.

8

SHORT-LIVED THOUGHTS

These are the light pieces of your mental health equipment – the ones you can pick up and put down with ease. Lots of repetition is pretty easy with these, and you are unlikely to get injured using them. They pop into your mind, don't take up too much space and then disappear. It's not that they don't have an impact – on the contrary, this type of thinking is what happens when we brainstorm and build great ideas – but they are generally quite malleable and may just be the products of your mind bouncing around and experimenting with new viewpoints and how new information fits together; the 'what-ifs', 'I wonders' and 'do you thinks . . .' all come into this category. We can usually take or leave short-lived thoughts without too much tension.

LONG-LIVED THOUGHTS

These are the pieces of equipment we carry around with us. They are a bit heavier and they develop and are repeated over time, tending to be reinforced through life experiences, which is how they make their gains. Long-lived thoughts are more like wearing a weighted vest or ankle straps than the equipment you can pick up and put down. The weight of them can change over time and they are harder to shift. Indeed, we want these weights to be helpful and actively make you stronger, rather than weighing you down. They can be adjusted though, and yes, you guessed it – they make for heavier work than your short-lived thoughts.

INTRUSIVE THOUGHTS

Both short- and long-lived thoughts can cause us trouble if we don't know how to use our equipment. Short-lived thoughts can pick up too much pace and leave us feeling out of control, while long-lived thoughts have the potential to become too heavy to carry around and start to cause us pain. Unchecked, short-lived thoughts can turn into fear, negative self-talk, rumination and resentment, while long-lived thoughts can turn into shame-based core beliefs about yourself and the world. When this happens, we call these thoughts intrusive.

Intrusive thoughts are the equivalent of using equipment that is far too fast and heavy, creating a risk of injury. Usually unpleasant and a bit of a shock when we notice them, they most often occur when we feel psychologically threatened, internally or externally, and our minds start preparing for the worst-case scenario by picking up the heaviest and most intense piece of equipment available.

Intrusive thoughts are, in fact, an extremely normal part of the human experience. But because we don't talk about them much, they can often be judged as mad, bad or sad, and are considered socially undesirable. Through our silence, they gather momentum as we keep them secret, feel ashamed and attach significance to them by allowing them to mean something negative about who we are, judging ourselves in exactly the way we fear and attempt to avoid in others. Intrusive thoughts have the potential to become a long-lived narrative that we carry around.

JOURNAL OPPORTUNITY
Do you have any thoughts, intrusive or otherwise,
that you'd like to acknowledge at this point?

Take a minute, in private, to write them down. As we
work through the programme, you may spot themes,
patterns and changes that allow the charge to come out of
any intrusive thoughts that might block your progress.
This is the very start of you noticing your patterns and
identifying your individual process.

- -

- -

Feelings

For the purposes of this book, I will use the terms 'feelings'
and 'mental health muscle' interchangeably.

This is where the magic happens. Because feelings are
literally energy in your body. They are the sensations you
feel when something happens: your heart dropping when
you get some bad news, butterflies in your tummy when you
are nervous or in love, feeling rooted to the spot or frozen
when you are scared, that tight feeling in your chest and
your heart speeding up. It's these physical experiences that
inform you of how you are feeling.

Lots of us try to *think* about how we feel, rather than *feel* about it, but the truth is, you cannot think your feelings. You have to feel them. We all have them; they are always there. And whether you work on them or not is totally up to you. I will tell you this, however: if you want to grow and heal, you have to work on your feelings. As a therapist, I have witnessed many people try to overcome psychological and emotional pain while still trying to avoid their feelings. In the long run, it does not work.

Feelings are what help us communicate; they are how we influence each other's energy, and they are in control of our body language, which conveys our truth with much more speed than our thoughts can, whether that is our intention or not. They motivate our behaviours and when we are attuned to them, they can help us through important events without us having to think every little detail through. The more intense feelings also support us to overcome major obstacles in life like loss, rejection and trauma. Feelings are our journey – they are what move us from anger, denial, shame and guilt into acceptance, letting go and mindfulness. They are signals and indications that something is happening, whether that thing is good, bad, passive or dangerous. Feelings will be used as a call to action throughout the programme.

As discussed, we've conveniently given words to some of the most common sensations and feelings, turning them into communicable thoughts. When our equipment (thoughts) and our muscle (feelings) are working well together, we feel at ease, but when they jar, are in conflict or we don't know how to help ourselves, our mental health suffers.

During my time as a therapist, I have come across hundreds

of super-smart people who have the capacity and competence to think their way around anything. Yet, they are left muddled because they cannot think themselves through or out of their feelings. I often hear people in sessions say, 'I feel stuck; I just want to get over it'. What this usually means is exactly what it suggests: that they want to step *over* their feelings, rather than feel *through* them. But stepping over them does not unstick them. Only working through them does.

We feel anxious and stressed when we try to think our way out of our feelings because we don't stop thinking for long enough for our feelings to catch up and unstick us. This is the 'doing' rather than 'being' syndrome. Think about it: if we ignored physical sensations when we moved muscles in our bodies, we wouldn't know how to make ourselves comfortable or challenge our muscles to work harder. We have to pay attention to our feelings in the same way because they inform the mind of its next move.

Within therapy, with most clients, there is a session or two (or more) when feelings come to the surface and we get to really see what's going on emotionally. Feelings are powerful and can take over involuntarily. It is often these moments that allow us to build a fundamental understanding and compassion for ourselves. Sometimes we call it an emotional detox and it looks different on everyone; it is not necessarily a breakdown or lots of crying – it can be more subtle that that. It clears the mind and allows your mental health muscle to relax and release.

Feeling in order to heal means you stop ignoring or avoiding feelings; instead, you invite them in fully and, eventually, integrate them as part of your health journey.

There are seven foundation feelings that I was taught about and that I like to focus on:

Feelings	Related to:	The sensation you might feel:
Joy	Hope, relief, happiness, excitement, gratitude, satisfaction, playfulness, contentment, pride, peacefulness, optimism, calm, gladness, inspired	A light feeling all over the body; a sense of bounciness, smiling
Love	Affection, desire, compassion, arousal, passion, respect, trust, empathy, acceptance, caring	A warm swelling in your chest area; power and energy in your body, as well as sexual arousal
Anger	Resentment, annoyance, irritation, frustration, fury, rage, hate, outrage, impatience, agitation, assertiveness, sarcasm, crankiness, aggravation	An energetic feeling all over your body; clenching your fists, headaches, fatigue, frowning
Pain	Sadness, loneliness, hurt, pity, hopelessness, pressure, grief, heartbreak, home-sickness, abandonment, betrayal, being down, burdened, jealous	A pain in your lower chest and/or heart; actual physical pain, welling up behind your eyes, a knot in your gut

Shame	Embarrassment, humility, exposed, worthlessness, icky, dirtiness, nausea, humiliation, stigmatised, criticised, envy, rejection	Your face, neck and chest might feel hot, a sick feeling in your tummy, wanting to hide away, not being able to make eye contact
Fear	Apprehension, overwhelm, threatened, scared, nervous, doubt, horror, worry, bravery, panic, powerlessness, helplessness	A tingling sensation, tightness in your extremities or chest, butterflies in your tummy
Guilt	Regret, blame, bad, remorse, apologetic, sorry	Eroding sensation in your abdomen, twitchiness in your hands, the bottom of your feet feeling heavy or stuck

As you can see from the table above, most other feelings are variations of intensity within these seven. For example, things like frustration, irritation and feeling annoyed fit into the anger category; gratitude, excitement and satisfaction fit into the joy category. And so on.

Over the next five weeks, I have no doubt you will have to work with most, if not all, of these foundation feelings. In the physio section of this book (see pp.197–216), you will find a selection of exercises to support you in managing these, along with stress, letting go, rejection, control and hope. I have also included some specific mental health workouts for anxiety, obsession, compulsion, depression and self-sabotage for anyone who experiences these.

I know – you are probably realising that this is going to be quite hard work? And I agree; feelings are hard work. Lots of us like the idea of but do not really enjoy the experience of being attuned to our feelings and taking the time to go slowly enough to allow them to inform us about who we are and what we need. I include myself in that. When I am really, honestly, authentically working on my feelings, I am often very uncomfortable, particularly if I am with someone else like my therapist or significant other. For me, it is being witnessed in my feelings that is most challenging – we will talk more about this soon.

MENTAL HEALTH MYTH

'Feeling means suffering'

Often, the thing that gets us in a muddle about feelings is that when we start to feel, we confuse the unease we experience with suffering.

Feeling is alleviating and cathartic; it does not mean you will suffer. Suffering happens as a result of your thinking and perspective on a given situation. For example, if you tell yourself that every time you do a push-up it is going to hurt, the likelihood is that your mind will interpret it as suffering and something to move away from. Whereas if every time you do a push-up you tell yourself you are getting stronger, your mind is likely to find the exercise more invigorating than painful. Until you can reposition your thoughts and feel the feelings as they come, you might well feel like you are suffering. As your perspective changes, so will the way you think and feel about things.

Feelings will not injure you. It is the *avoidance* of feelings that allows you to behave ignorantly, dishonestly, passively. Throughout this programme, we will help your mind to learn that feelings are helpful. We will be gathering evidence that feelings and the sense of vulnerability that comes with having them, are not a failing, nor do they make you a victim of suffering. Again, they are that call to action, and they create hope and emotional resilience.

It is our feelings – our mental health muscle – that help us to make changes and, furthermore, good decisions in life. They are, as I said, our energy, our charge, and my belief is that the world would be a happier and more harmonious place if we were all given permission to consider our feelings more honestly and had some guidance on how to handle them appropriately.

All that being said, it is important to understand that using the workouts here won't mean being able to get rid of feelings or even control them. It will mean that you will know what to do when they happen and have a choice about how you behave in response. You gain this kind of resilience by taking the opportunity to experience your feelings, working with them and being interested in what they are trying to tell you.

We are all born with the natural capacity to handle our own feelings – and taking yourself to that place can be a challenge and yes, a little scary, because it is new, and you may feel suspicious of where it will lead. We are starting to bring your psychological edges into view and it is what you choose to do at your edges that makes a difference. You get to decide whether you need to sharpen or smooth them. If this was a physical workout, this would be where the change happens – where the muscle starts adapting to a new form of movement. And your mental health muscle is the same. Whenever you hear me talk about feelings or working with them, you can imagine you are right at that point in your workout where you can accept the challenge . . . or not. The challenge is there to improve strength and endurance around your mental health muscle.

Each time you learn how to work with feelings and how they connect with yourself, translating them into healthy thoughts and behaviours, you are increasing your range of (e-)motion for a happy, healthy and curious mind.

Behaviour

Behaviour is where both we and others see our mental health strengths and limitations, vulnerabilities and developments.

Behaviour is evidence of your hard work. It is the things you choose to do, or not do. You are ultimately responsible and accountable for all these choices. There will be significant changes in your thoughts and feelings as we move through the next five weeks, but the first and most obvious results will be in your behaviours.

Sometimes our behaviour makes objective sense and sometimes it can seem strange to the outsider, particularly when we are in a state of transition. When we are too much in our thoughts or, indeed, feelings, internal conflict develops, meaning that we are effectively forced to start behaving in ways that attempt to balance us back out. This internal conflict is usually a result of trying to avoid feelings and a bid to hold on to an existing belief system or long-lived thoughts. We call this psychological conflict 'cognitive dissonance'.

If you were exercising while physically injured and unable to appropriately use a specific muscle group, your body would start to compensate in other areas to make the movement you are attempting possible. This is risky as it can cause further damage to other muscle groups. Well, guess what? Your mind does the same thing. The mind seeks consistency, congruence and balance. We know that maximum change happens when we are consistent, and we also know that it can be very hard to remain consistent in a behaviour if it does not balance well with our thoughts and feelings. In fact, it can cause increased levels of stress. The dissonant space – or tension – that is created between our thoughts, feelings and behaviours is a psychological danger zone, as it can mean that we are dodging emotion through underuse of our mental health muscle (feelings), while overusing our mental health equipment (thoughts) to rationalise behaviours that do not align with our core values. Internal conflict and tension increase and the mind will start to compensate for this discomfort in an attempt to ease it, rejecting any change we try to make through unconsciously forcing us back into more familiar patterns and behaviours.

The return to old behaviours and compensations can appear quite similar to each other; they look like anxiety, perfectionism, disordered eating, addictions, depressive thoughts, seeking external validation, attacking others, attacking self, a lack of motivation and a desire to isolate. You may also recognise others that you can add to this list. The behaviours described here are often not optional because they have developed through less conscious attempts to cope and survive and, occasionally, they feel like your only option. For example, if your core belief is that you are worth less than other people, then when you attempt to behave in a way that proves you are worthwhile, dissonance is created between what you think and how you behave and you'll experience unpleasant, tense feelings. Usually, when we get down to it, these feelings can be named as shame or rage. Over the next five weeks, you will be working in a dissonant space and it will be uncomfortable. The difference now, however, will be that you are choosing to make that transition – you are choosing to work at your psychological edge in order to evoke positive change. If you feel unable to manage these feelings, you might find yourself behaving in a way that proves you are worth less once more, so that the tension (the feelings – the dissonance) go away and you get to continue to live in the belief that you are worth less than other people.

Carrying around equipment like this feels heavy for you and those around you and brings your mood down, which can start to feel like depression. This programme will help you to use this very human process and all the feelings involved to align your thoughts, feelings and behaviours and support you to work with them until everything matches up. Once you are more conscious of this process playing out, you will find it easier to be consistent and generally feel a bit happier, as you start to create more choices for the good of your mental health, putting in the necessary measures before it takes a tumble. (If this is a new concept to you, you may need to reread this paragraph a couple of times.)

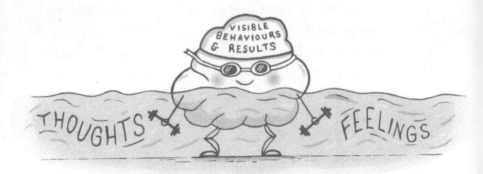

You cannot see this type of healing and change, so you have to be extra patient. Your mental health heals in private and strengthens slowly, so that it can then give you long-term stability, flexibility and strength to create the internal backdrop you need in order to function within an external worlds you feel satisfied with.

Let's talk about genetics

Something we do not explicitly cover in this book are the genetics involved in mental health. Indeed, mental health is, in part, genetic – but that does not mean you are not responsible for looking after your mind. I consider it helpful to acknowledge the genetics involved, but to focus on them as reasons for problems runs the risk of making excuses. In fact, many a time, I have worked with people who come from a long line of mental health suffering and when they start to make changes for themselves – taking responsibility and being accountable and committed to the process of looking after the integrity of their minds – that line of suffering comes to an end. Maybe, just maybe, that is you!

Before we go any further, take this moment to cement why you are doing this at this point in your life. Write it down, so you don't lose sight of your 'why'.

 JOURNAL OPPORTUNITY: WHY NOW?

When we understand why we are doing something we are far more inclined to stick with it. Are you doing this because you enjoy it? Has a life event led you to want to take better care of your emotional health? Have you identified unhelpful psychological patterns? Are you fed up with sabotaging yourself? Is your psychological wellbeing the missing link in your health journey? If you answer 'yes' to these or any other questions or statements that come up for you, you can use this as your 'why'. Each time you come to a tricky spot and question why you are bothering to embark on such a major challenge, come back to your 'why', your intention. It will help you stay motivated, even when your willpower is at its lowest.

- -

- -

Chapter 2

GOAL SETTING

MOTIVATION IS SOMETHING you are going to need throughout the next five weeks, and one of the best ways to maintain stamina and endurance around this is to set realistic goals for yourself.

When we set goals, we ignite hope within ourselves, which, in turn, helps to build psychological resilience. Think of it as your active recovery period: it's all about how you bounce back when you get tired or burnt out. People who have realistic goals in their sights tend to recover quicker when something unhelpful happens or they come off the programme for some reason.

I must stress that your mental health goals should be realistic and timely, so that you can feel positive about your mental health journey, and not just about the end product. Setting realistic and timely goals is more difficult for some than for others because, while they can help to maintain motivation, they also draw attention to where you are right now. And depending on how you feel about your current circumstances, it can sometimes feel painful to acknowledge that where you are is not where you want to be. It is important to remember to use those difficult feelings as a call to action, to motivate you to move forward, up and out, rather than holding you back and bringing you down.

Setting Mental Health Goals

There are five things your mental health goals should do:

- Get you motivated
- Open your mind
- Allow for mistakes
- Leave room for improvement
- Stabilise your mood

How to Set Your Goals

1. Consider where you want to be five weeks from now. For example: *happier, healthier, more resilient, more connected, with stronger boundaries, good self-esteem and I want to experience fewer mood swings.*

2. What do you think you need to target to get there? For example: *I need to target my self-esteem order to feel stronger, my loneliness in order to build connection, my anxiety to level out my mood.*

3. Ensure your chosen target motivates and inspires you to take action. *Check in with how you feel when you*

think about this goal; if it motivates you, move on to the next step. If it does not, then create a 'future goals' list and pop it in there for now. You'll be amazed how many more things you'll feel motivated by once we get your motivation activated . . .

4. Write down your goals. And stick with them! *Don't move the goalposts as you go – that only leads to problems with perfectionism. If you feel you have achieved your goal, set a brand new one (or pick one from you 'future goals' list), and consider the old one completed.*

5. Align your internal and external environment with your goals. *Research tells us that how we set ourselves up when working towards and achieving our goals is like any type of sport, where we'd have the correct gear and the right location sorted. Our minds need that too. Align your external world by ensuring you have the social support you need and any practical points organised like removing or providing a particular thing. Align your internal world by ensuring you are speaking to yourself in the right ways and making changes with the intention of self-care. This programme will help you do all these things incrementally, so don't worry if it sounds difficult right now.*

My suggestion is always to start with one. Just one goal. The one you want or need most. You may have some others in your sights, and you can put them in your 'future goals' list. If you feel overwhelmed, it's highly probable (actually, scientifically proven) that you are much less likely to stay committed. And on that note, be prepared to recommit to your goal on average once a month, as lapses in action and commitment are a very typical and normal part of this process.

JOURNAL OPPORTUNITY: WRITE DOWN YOUR GOALS

Write your first mental health goal down and create space for 'future goals' if you like that idea. It can also be helpful, and part of setting up good external support, to share your goal with someone you trust.

You should now have a clear understanding of why you are embarking on Your Mental Health Workout, what you'd like to change and where you'd like to be five weeks from now.

_ _

_ _

Congratulations on getting to this point. You now have the foundations and information you need to move into the main event. Feel free at any point to come back to these first chapters for reference, underline the bits you relate to or want to memorise, and even the bits that don't entirely make sense to you just yet. Hold on to the sparks of inspiration and motivation you felt as you were reading and let's now move into getting you psychologically warmed up.

PART TWO

YOUR MENTAL HEALTH WORKOUT

YOUR MENTAL HEALTH WORKOUT

5 WEEKS TO A HEALTHIER, HAPPIER MIND

WARM UP:

CREATING AND KEEPING SELF-ESTEEM, THE CORE STABILITY TO YOUR MENTAL HEALTH. PLUS EXPLORATION OF YOUR RANGE OF MOTION, MADE UP OF YOUR BOUNDARIES AND VULNERABILITY.

WEEKLY WORKOUTS:

1 X THERAPUTIC SPACE
2 X SOCIAL EVENTS
3 X EXERCISE
4 X SELF-CARE

DAILY WORKOUTS:

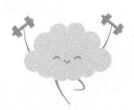

1 X MINDFULNESS
2 X CONNECTION
3 X APPRECIATION
4 X MOVEMENT

Come back to this quick reference guide throughout the programme to remind you of the various elements of our workout metaphor.

FEELINGS = YOUR MENTAL HEALTH MUSCLE

THOUGHTS = YOUR MENTAL HEALTH WORKOUT EQUIPMENT

BEHAVIOUR = RESULTS

CORE STABILITY = SELF-ESTEEM

BOUNDARIES + VULNERABILITY = RANGE OF MOTION

THERAPEUTIC SPACES = YOUR MENTAL HEALTH PERSONAL TRAINER

SOCIAL EVENTS = TECHNIQUE CHECK-IN

EXERCISE = LITERALLY CARDIOVASCULAR EXERCISE

SELF-CARE = FUEL AND NUTRITION

MINDFULNESS = HYDRATION

CONNECTION = AEROBIC WORKOUT

APPRECIATION = THE FINISHER

MOVEMENT = YOUR COOLDOWN

Chapter 3

WARMING UP - CORE STABILITY AND RANGE OF MOTION

⎯ ⎯ ⎯ ⎯

AS WITH ANY type of workout, the first thing we need to do is to get the muscle groups we'll be targeting warmed up and mobile. This provides you with a solid foundation and reduces your risk of injury. For your mental health, the main muscle groups that need activating are your self-esteem (core stability) and your boundaries and vulnerability (your psychological range of motion).

Self-esteem

Self-esteem means we feel aligned, balanced, equal and worthy of love.

Our self-esteem tells us how we feel about ourselves and affects pretty much everything we do; it is a very intimate experience, and it exists at the core of our being. Hence, it is the core-stability workout for our mental health.

As with any other workout, the first thing we have to do is get the muscle group we are targeting activated. So let's start on the next page with simply activating and mobilising the basic idea around self-esteem: that you can accept who you are, just as you are, right now, in this moment.

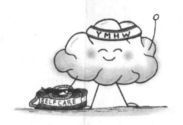

MOBILISING YOUR
CORE STABILITY

An observation exercise

1: Look in the mirror each morning and evening and simply observe what you see. Notice where your attention falls and what happens in your thinking and your feelings. You may notice some uncomfortable twinges in your mental health muscle around the things you see that you do not like about yourself. Work with this. Stay with it. Do not pass judgment. You may also, in time, not only observe your physical body but find that this exercise also connects you with what's happening inside too.

2: Fill in the gaps in the sentence below and repeat, either to yourself or out loud, three times:

'I notice I feel _____ about my _____ and I accept myself anyway.'

Any anxiety that arises as a result of the above exercise is to be gently worked with. We are just mobilising and activating your core stability, so go carefully with yourself when applying this. Start small, and as you practise, you will naturally progress into the interaction between self-acceptance and self-esteem.

When you feel you are ready, move on to the full workout progression.

Note: I will be using the terms core stability and self-esteem interchangeably throughout this workout.

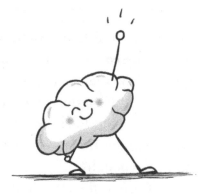

CORE-STABILITY WORKOUT

1: Introduce stabilising movements

A stabilising movement is an action that encapsulates everything we have discussed so far. It is about working with your mental health muscle, being responsible and doing the next most loving thing for your mental health.

Ask yourself: what can I do today that allows me to be responsible and accepting towards myself and gives me the message that I am good enough?

When you answer this question, remember your core is not just your abdominal muscles – it includes loads of other little muscles at the front and back of your body. And your self-esteem is the same: varied 'movements', like having commitments, helping others, standing up for what you believe in and doing it, regardless of what the chatter in your mind is telling you about yourself – these are all ways to activate your core stability.

2: Create stabilising thoughts

Through initiating stabilising movements, you offer yourself the message that you are aligned, balanced, equal and worthy. In most cases, your stabilising thoughts will organically follow on from that.

Stabilising thoughts come in two forms: thoughts that anchor and soothe you and thoughts that give you positive and motivating messages.

Take some time now to write down three thoughts that soothe you:

1.

2.

3.

And three thoughts that are positive and motivating to you:

1.

2.

3.

Excuse anything that comes up that does not feel stabilising; just let it pass. Thoughts and behaviour tend to organically improve the more you do this exercise.

These two exercises work in tandem. Sometimes we have to create stabilising thoughts so that, in turn, we are able to feel good enough to show up for ourselves in a healthier way; and sometimes we have to introduce stabilising movements first, so that we find that we start to believe good enough things about ourselves and the stabilising thoughts create themselves along the way. Take some time to experiment and see what works best for you.

3: Maintenance

The third step is simply repetition. Because variation and consistency are key. Do this warm-up exercise as often as possible and in as many different areas of your life as you can to keep that core stability in really good shape.

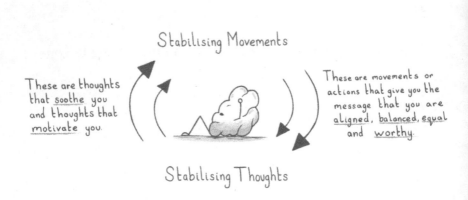

Stabilising Movements

These are thoughts that soothe you and thoughts that motivate you.

These are movements or actions that give you the message that you are aligned, balanced, equal and worthy.

Stabilising Thoughts

WHY WE DO THIS WORKOUT

In the previous chapters, we laid some excellent groundwork, helping you to understand your mental health and set your mental health goals, ready for action. We talked about 'foundation feelings', the different parts of your mental health muscle, and via this core-stability warm-up you will become familiar with what it feels like to be working out each part of that muscle.

Most of us, at times, find our core stability isn't quite where we want it to be. With your core stability out of shape, everything else feels a bit more problematic. It is your ultimate support system – your powerhouse – and without it, you are more prone to injury, which, in terms of your mental health, will show up as increased anxiety, feelings of failure and potentially a loss of purpose. Many of the people I have worked with have had trouble understanding that their core stability needs working on because the compensations they previously used to make them feel stronger in this department – for example, external validation or instant gratification – have worked effectively for an extended period of time. If you are already experiencing anxiety, depression, helplessness and hopelessness, we know that your core is not supporting you in the way it should.

When your core is off balance, you never get the chance to familiarise yourself with your level of capability, standards, values or motives; you will be constantly working above or below where you actually need to be, rather than within your own range of motion. You will feel less inclined to develop the motivation needed to be consistent in looking after or respecting yourself. Hence, it is important to figure out what your core stability looks and feels like and how to engage it.

We work on our self-esteem because it affects the results we want for ourselves and the choices we make about how to get them. At this very early point in the programme, whatever state your mental health muscle and equipment are in and whatever the results you crave, just take this time to know that after all is said and done, nothing is more important than how you feel and what you think about yourself; if you only stick to one thing during your first week of the programme, let it be this core-stability workout.

All the things you think and feel, along with every behaviour you engage in, are ultimately your responsibility, and coming back to your core workout affirms your ability and willingness to be accountable at the most fundamental of levels. Taking responsibility is a good thing, by the way! It means that you get to be in charge of your own life, yourself, your thoughts, feelings and behaviours. We tend to like that idea. The muddle we sometimes get into is when we realise that taking responsibility also means being prepared to accept the consequences for our thoughts, feelings and behaviours, choices and mistakes, good and bad.

We can sometimes confuse the idea of taking responsibility with making ourselves available to take the blame for things and in a worst-case scenario, shame too. If our belief system misguidedly holds on to the idea that we don't want to take responsibility for our real or perceived failures, we also cannot feel fully responsible for our hard work and our successes. When we do not take responsibility for ourselves, we reinforce disempowering and negative feelings and thoughts about ourselves and feel like victims. This generates an undesirable internal and external experience. And this is why we work on core stability first; this is how what you think of you is created, which is great news, because it means you also have the power to change it.

The other fundamental reason for working on self-esteem is that it can change, depending on where you are and who you are around, and it is really important that you are familiar with which areas of your life you have sturdy self-esteem in and which you do not. No one, not even those of us with psychology qualifications and therapeutic backgrounds, have perfectly balanced core stability the whole time. I will draw on the physical comparison again here: even if you were (or are) a professional athlete, you would have days, times and circumstances that leave you a bit off balance and feeling not quite as steady, fast and strong. A runner who does a long run one day may find that they are a bit wobbly in their strength training the next, for example, even though it doesn't take away from their overall fitness level. Likewise, following a hit to your self-esteem, you may notice an effect on your ability to stay aligned and balanced in the moment and, potentially, for a while afterwards.

SELF-ESTEEM WOBBLES

Most of us are aware that the feeling of not being good enough is an issue and stops us fulfilling our potential and giving 100 per cent in life. But did you also know that a sense or feeling that you are better than others is also an indication that your core stability is out of shape? And it has similar effects. Feeling 'better than' others shows up in how we think. For example, 'I have better shoes than him' or 'I am more intelligent than her'. You might also notice yourself swinging from one end to the other: 'Oh my, she is so beautiful. But actually, I am smarter, wealthier and better than her in other ways.' Thinking, feeling and behaving as if you are worth more or less than anyone else are core-stability wobbles, and this workout should encourage a feeling of balance and stability within your relationship with yourself.

CORE STABILITY

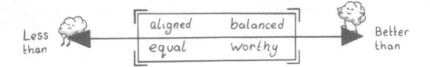

The above diagram indicates how large the 'equal' area is for us all. There's loads of space to manoeuvre around our strengths and limitations before we fall off the ends into less than or better than and have a self-esteem wobble.

Strong self-esteem means you are able to take responsibility for yourself entirely, without blaming, shaming or judging anyone, including yourself, along the way. You can acknowledge your strengths and limitations without feeling as if they change your fundamental value as a person, and when you do so, you will still like yourself. That is what getting in shape looks like. When your core stability kicks in, you will feel aligned, balanced, equal and worthy. The wobbles are always useful, however, because they tell you where the work is, so do pay attention to them as you do your core-stability workout.

HOW TO GET THIS WORKOUT WORKING FOR YOU

Getting to understand the nuances of your psychological core stability is how you train yourself to understand your patterns and start to pre-empt where you might need more work, help and support. So you might notice, for example, that you feel very balanced at home with your family, while you tend to feel off balance at work. In this case, we can see that you are able to feel aligned, balance, equal and worthy with your family, so we know your core has the capacity to support you in this way. But we need to help you transfer some of that strength into other areas, such as your work life, social events or when you are alone.

In which areas of your life do you feel aligned, balanced, equal and worthy? In which areas of your life do you feel wobbly, unbalanced, unequal and unworthy?

What you are identifying here are the areas of your life in which your core stability is strong and where it is not. Where you feel strong, it is likely because the external circumstances support you well. Family, hobbies, work and social media are just some of the most common examples that might come up. We label this 'external stability' because it comes in from the outside. It is useful to have and know about and is a bit like borrowing gym equipment that helps make you stronger or watching someone else do the move, so you can copy it – both great ways of getting a workout working for you. But guess what? That equipment (and thinking) will always belong to someone else. If you rely on external events entirely, when your primary source of stability is no longer available, anxiety thrives and your mental health suffers. You need to know how to create and maintain your 'internal stability', so you can support yourself too.

JOURNAL OPPORTUNITY: TAKE A FEW MINUTES TO THINK AND WRITE ABOUT THE INTERNAL EVENTS THAT AFFECT YOUR CORE STABILITY

These are things that come from inside you and don't need an external event to trigger them. For example, when I feel tired, I tend to feel a bit sad and sorry for myself and am a bit off balance; or when I remember what it was like to be bullied at school, I feel unworthy and full of shame. I know this comes from the inside because it is not actually happening right now.

_ _

_ _

Having read through the core-stability workout and the why-we-do-it and how-to-get-it-working-for-you sections, you might be cultivating an awareness of some of the unhelpful habits you've picked up that need attention. Everyone's unhelpful habits are slightly different, so let's try an exercise to explore what you might need to address.

UNHELPFUL HABITS IN RELATION TO SELF-ESTEEM

These are often rooted in negative core beliefs about yourself. Do you recognise any of the following?

- No one likes me.
- I am unlovable.
- I am a bad person.
- I am stupid.
- I am ugly.
- I'm not good enough.
- I'm not worth it.
- I am boring.
- People are not interested in me.
- I do not have an impact.
- I can't change.

When you find a negative core belief you identify with, ask yourself the following questions:

- In what situation is it most likely to come up?
- What effect does this have on my feelings?
- What effect does this have on my thoughts?
- What effect does this have on my behaviour?
- What previous life experience has contributed to the development of this core belief?

List three pieces of evidence that challenge the negative core belief or reinforce a positive one.

1.

2.

3.

Challenging our core beliefs and working on our core stability is a big workout, so if the questions above feel too overwhelming right now, modify by simply saying the exact opposite of your negative belief to yourself three times in a row for a week and see what shifts. Then you can come back to the list of questions in a more specific way.

We are off to a great start. Anything you do from hereon in that is related to Your Mental Health Workout will, in some way, be working on your core stability. Just like your abdominal muscles, if you work on your self-esteem each day, it is a part of you that can strengthen quickly. Then, once you've got it in the shape you like, and it is strong enough to hold together who you are – even during challenging and unprecedented times – you can choose to move on to a more personalised maintenance programme beyond these first five weeks in which you pick the parts that work for you and integrate them into your life to help you keep up your desired results.

Boundaries and Vulnerability: Your Psychological Range of Motion

As you start to feel more aligned, balanced, equal and worthy following the previous workout, you'll notice that your desire to progress and adapt how you use your core stability naturally leads you to changes in how you activate your mental strength and flexibility – namely, your boundaries and vulnerability. Together, these make up your psychological range of motion – or (e-)motion.

In this workout, we will explore how your boundaries and vulnerability work together to protect the integrity of your mind, making you feel defined on the inside and on the outside.

Note:

1. You have authority over the intensity and strength of any boundary you explore.

2. You have the right to change their intensity at any point.

MOBILISING YOUR RANGE OF MOTION WORKOUT

1. Set yourself up by reading the information in this section and use it to help you identify the strength and flexibility improvements you'd like to make. Include these in your mental health goals.

2. Can you identify a specific example of when your range of motion, your boundaries and vulnerability, were not where you needed them to be? For example, I notice that I find it difficult to say 'no' to people at work, or I that I feel way too vulnerable when I talk about my mental health with my friends.

3. What feelings do you have that inform you of this – do you tense up, feel angry, shocked, lose your voice, shut down?

Once you have mobilised and actively considered your psychological range of motion via asking yourself the above three questions, move on to the full workout.

Range-of-motion workout

1. IDENTIFY THE BOUNDARY THAT NEEDS SETTING.
You can use one you identified in the mobilisation exercise above.

2. IMAGINE WHAT IT IS THAT YOU WOULD LIKE TO SAY OR DO IN ORDER TO SET THIS BOUNDARY. You don't have to do it on the spot, straight away. Imagine and practise it in your own time and in your own mind, so that when the opportunity arises you feel able to put it into action. Doing this helps take the charge and intensity out of any feelings that have informed this boundary, and therefore going over it in private will help you to manage your vulnerability in the situation.

Note: please remember that boundaries are about intimacy, vulnerability and connection; they are about love and self-respect.

3. BE BRAVE AND SET THE BOUNDARY. Once you've practised what you want to say, with love, go back to the situation/person you need the boundary with and speak/action it.

4. FEEL THE FEELINGS AND HOLD THE BOUNDARY. You will feel vulnerable and you will feel all the things you don't want to feel. Your job here is to hold your position – that's how your range of (e-)motion adjusts, and it is probably the hardest part!

5. REPEAT – as necessary.

WHY WE DO THIS WORKOUT

In physical fitness, range of motion is a phrase used to describe the amount of movement a joint can tolerate in active, passive or combination exercises. This means you need both strength and flexibility to be involved. Generally speaking, we seek to increase a range of motion that is too small, maintain a range of motion that is safe and healthy and contain a range of motion that is too large in order to keep the muscle group healthy, useful and active. We do this through flexibility and strength training. Your mind works in a similar way.

Our psychological range of motion is largely dependent on our life experiences. It is a learned mechanism that we inherit from the role models around us. If we are lucky enough to have stable, solid and secure attachments to healthy role models, that's great. However, because of the historical stigma attached to getting help with our minds, many of us have been raised by parents who did not have access to this information or, indeed, the freedom to seek help, and who therefore passed on unhelpful habits and behaviours, through no fault of their own.

We are taught implicitly, and in some cases explicitly, that academics, beauty or creative education and endeavours are more significant than the condition of our minds. With parents often feeling under-skilled and challenged, it can feel simpler to leave this very important work around boundaries and vulnerability and how they can be helpful, along with loving acts of self-care, to replacement attachment figures such as teachers or peers, whom they know little about. As a result, most adults who come to my consulting room are surprised to hear about the concept of boundaries and unsure or even resistant to the benefits of vulnerability.

At some point in our lives, every single one of us will be confronted with the need to work on our boundaries. If you have too small or too large a range of motion, it is highly likely that your core stability will take the hit, leaving you feeling out of shape and lacking definition, having to compensate through external validation and instant gratification. You will have self-esteem wobbles, and without the appropriate stretching and strengthening – i.e. coping mechanisms – these wobbles are difficult to bounce back from and you may feel you have to start from scratch again. We do this workout to experiment with our boundaries and find out where we need them to be.

Just like your body, your mind enjoys feeling healthy, defined, strong and flexible. Without a healthy psychological range of motion, you have no choice but to reject your feelings and your truth goes into hiding. You find it difficult to know who you are and how to define yourself; consequently, you have difficulties in relationships with yourself and others. You lose yourself – and feeling lost is one of the scariest physical and psychological experiences human beings can have. This workout ensures that you no longer have to shut down or overextend yourself in order to people-please, get what you think you want, feel gratified and find validation or love solely in the eyes of others. This workout gives you a choice about how you move and how you define yourself, rather than sticking to the specific set of rules you've learned from your role models or society. It helps you to know who you are and supports you in learning or relearning what is a healthy range of motion for you. This warm-up workout will also inform the intensity with which you apply the weekly and daily ones.

This is very personal work. I have never worked with two clients who have the same range of motion; therefore, this is also the therapeutic work that often energises me the most because I really get to know and understand who a person is. It is also, very often, a turning point in therapy: when you learn what it means to have boundaries – setting and holding them while exploring vulnerability – you take ultimate responsibility for your mental health.

WHY ARE BOUNDARIES AND VULNERABILITY PART OF THE SAME WORKOUT?

Good question! Boundaries and vulnerability might seem like opposing concepts, but they are, in fact, psychological movements that have a direct effect on each other. Both are emotionally challenging and intimate and require strength of mind and heart to engage with. We absolutely need to be able to exercise authority over how vulnerable we feel, and boundaries help us to do that. Anyone who has ever experienced emotional pain, such as a feeling of being rejected or a real or perceived failure, will know exactly why this is important. Knowing how to use your psychological range of motion is a bit like knowing when to go all out in the gym, when to take it easy and when to have a rest day: vulnerability informs us of our needs, then boundaries allow us to take appropriate action.

As we are practising listening to your feelings here and

working with them, let me take this opportunity to point out that when experimenting with your range of motion, you will come up, once again, against some psychological edges. This is the equivalent to that feeling you get in a physical workout that makes you want to stop. Psychological edges are your current tolerance level – and there is a difference here: in a physical workout, you are often encouraged to push past your perceived limitations in order to get fitter and stronger. With your mind, however, you need to be gentler; yes, it is possible to explore and expand your edges via pushing yourself, but you also must be respectful of them. And the way to respect your edges is to notice if something feels good, cathartic and authentic. If you are able to hold on to the feeling of being aligned, balanced, equal and worthy that we created in the core-stability workout, you are usually on the right track and working out in a way that is good for your mind. If something kicks up self-doubt and you feel yourself backtracking into hiding or pain and shame that are intolerable or having self-esteem wobbles, that is a signal to change the form and technique of what you are doing and focus on the things that empower you (we will advance this further with social events on p. 83).

HOW TO GET THIS WORKOUT WORKING FOR YOU

Boundaries are your psychological strength. They protect your vulnerabilities, keeping you super-strong on the inside and creating definition that others can see on the outside, letting them know who you are. They are allowed to change over time.

There are two main categories of boundaries: visible and invisible. All this means is that there are different layers of strength being activated in different situations. We shall familiarise you with both, so that you know what is going to work for you – because they play out differently in everyone.

Eight things you need to know about boundaries

1. They allow for healthy intimacy.

2. They give you authority over your vulnerability.

3. They are an act of self-love and respect.

4. Boundary violations happen a lot.

5. It doesn't need to be like that.

6. You have the right to say yes and the right to say no.

7. You have the right to change your mind.

8. Boundaries create an opportunity to become intimate and vulnerable with yourself and others.

Visible boundaries

As their name suggests, these are boundaries, or layers of strength, that others can see. They include how physical you are with others and when, your personal space, what you say to others and also your sexual boundaries. Your skin is your first and foremost visible boundary. How you dress and use make-up could also be considered in this category.

Visible boundaries protect you from shame, trauma and resentment, via a life where you sit comfortably within your range of motion, not being pushed further than you can go. They let you deal with what is hurting you without hurting yourself. They are also a commitment to working with your feelings and not abandoning any part of you (see step 4 of the workout).

Visible boundaries are also the ones you set with friends, family members and colleagues, as well as with activities like how many times you go shopping per month or how much time you spend online.

Invisible boundaries

These denote the strength of self-love you hold for yourself. As discussed, you also learn this from your role models. It is likely that your invisible boundaries are similar to your role models', and if you've picked up unhelpful invisible boundaries from them, you can use exactly the same part of your mind to unlearn and relearn some helpful ones. Invisible boundaries help you tune into exactly who you are and stick to that, rather than attempting to define and love yourself through the eyes of others. This is an internal layer of strength that develops over time, allowing you to better align with your inner strength as an act of self-love. Generally speaking, these are felt; others cannot see them (hence 'invisible'). They support you to have faith in yourself, hold on to hope, help you to set limits within yourself, support yourself and also control what you allow into your internal experience.

You can have invisible boundaries within how you speak to yourself, how you care for yourself, what you believe in and the morals and values you hold for yourself.

 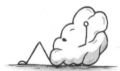

MENTAL HEALTH MYTHS

'Boundaries keep others away and are only necessary in an emergency – when we are angry with someone or need to reject someone'

Boundaries are entirely necessary for your close relationships. They help create definition inside and out, so that others know how to be in relationship with you. If you do any group exercise classes or share a gym space with others, you will be familiar with the idea of spacing out, so no one gets hurt. That is what we are doing here. Boundaries support your mental health by allowing you to identify your own feelings, thoughts and behaviours, even when emotionally challenged. They protect your core stability and create compassion and empathy for yourself and others. Boundaries tell people where you are at in this moment and invite them to be in relationship with you in a way that you can cope with.

'Boundaries are certain and cannot be changed once you put them in place'

Boundaries are malleable and changeable. They differ depending on changes in your internal and external world.

If your boundaries feel immovable, you are creating blocks and walls, not boundaries. Blocks and walls are only appropriate if the person you are setting boundaries with continues to push you and cause you pain. A bit like physical pain, sometimes we have to put a hard stop in if we are suddenly emotionally injured. Generally speaking though, strong and loving boundaries can be adjusted on the go and will still do the job.

> *'If I set boundaries, I am being selfish'*

We set boundaries to define who we are and create definition in our relationships. We take responsibility for ourselves when we set boundaries; there's a difference between being selfish and being self-centred!

> *'If I set boundaries, I'm going to be rejected'*

Boundaries are likely to cause disruption. The question is: if the backlash is that bad, why you were connected in the first place? If you cannot use the word 'no' in a relationship with yourself or others, then are you showing up as your true and best self? Clear boundaries allow for more love and more intimacy.

> *'Boundaries mean that I am angry'*

Boundaries are proactive, not reactive. People with strong boundaries experience less anger and fewer unwanted feelings. They do not allow themselves to be pushed around, and they have the strength to push back, so that they don't get hurt and angry about things. The boundary is a demonstration of love, not anger.

FLEXIBILITY

Understanding vulnerability as your psychological flexibility will help you get this workout working for you. Just like physical stretching, without regular consideration your mind stiffens up and creates pain and difficulty. Although working with your vulnerability can feel tender, I encourage it because, over time, if you do not stretch, you might *appear* super-tough and strong, yet in reality have a very limited range of emotional motion and have trouble setting boundaries and keeping your self-esteem in a place that is healthy for you. Ironically, *not* working with your vulnerability leaves your mental health tremendously vulnerable to further decline.

Look at it like this: if not stretching means you end up all stiff and tense and only able to move in one direction, and if taking risks involves trust, patience and courage, then allowing yourself to practise emotional strength and flexibility by being emotionally vulnerable is, in fact, a huge source of strength that can only serve to enhance your mental wellbeing. How do you do that? You feel your feelings! Any time your mental health muscle is activated and you are working with your feelings you have a chance to stretch out your vulnerability. Depending on what is going on around you and how you've used your mental health muscle recently, as well as on your history, culture and DNA, your psychological range of motion will differ from day to day, week to week and situation to situation.

I once worked with a client who told me he only did two feelings: 'fine' and 'angry'. He was a prime example of someone who had not been given the tools to safely explore his psychological flexibility and he used willpower to avoid his feelings or fire up his anger so that he appeared in control and looked strong and invulnerable on the outside. With some very close attention to what was happening in his internal world and carefully activating his flexibility and strength, where necessary, we were able to stretch out his vulnerability in a way that allowed him much more choice in life because he was then able to use his authority – his power – in a helpful way, rather than solely for avoidance or anger.

You might also find it helpful to identify the type of vulnerability you are working with. Is it physical (visible) or emotional (invisible)? Mostly here, we are talking about emotional vulnerabilities, but it is important to acknowledge that we have physical vulnerabilities too. For example, I have a physical vulnerability in my right wrist and when I push it too far, I feel pain. I have an emotional vulnerability around authority figures; I tend to worry about not being good enough and getting things wrong, which brings up feelings of fear and despair. I can work with both of these via my boundaries to keep me feeling safe, and it is also important that in order for both my wrist and my faith in myself to strengthen that I am exposed to these experiences.

Take a moment now to consider the connection here with visible and invisible boundaries. Put simply, as you become more familiar with the type of vulnerability you are working with and the feelings involved, you'll start to know what type of boundaries to work on. You'll practise exerting authority over the intensity of the feeling and using your internal strength (i.e. boundaries) to choose how and when you become vulnerable. The more authority you feel you have, the more variety and variations you'll have to choose from within your range-of-motion workout. As a side note, if this doesn't make sense to you just yet, don't worry – it is often very difficult to identify our own emotional vulnerabilities, as we are naturally protective and defensive around them. Just keep an eye out in the coming weeks for those raw moments where you can spot emotional vulnerability. Make a note of them in your journal.

I think it is particularly important to talk about how to get vulnerability working for you as the stigma around mental health in cultural groups and gender norms changes. Generally speaking, males have historically been shamed (more than females) for expressing feelings and vulnerability, and the shame around seeking therapeutic support lives on in particular cultures. So, yes, it is riskier for some than it is for others and can, in the first instance, feel more humiliating or raw to those who fall into certain social and cultural cohorts. Hence, this warm-up is vital for everyone – not only to expand your own range of motion, but also to help change how particular groups are stigmatised for expressing their mental health needs. When we understand that vulnerability and strength are what create a healthy psychological range of motion, we are able to give each other permission to find the strength within our vulnerability. The truth is that when it comes to vulnerability, there are no precise or exact answers. Just intuition, hope and giving yourself permission to trust the process.

Eight things you need to know about vulnerability

1. It allows you to keep your promises.

2. It is the essence of working with your feelings.

3. It allows you to stay in healthy relationships.

4. It looks after the health of your mind.

5. It keeps your conscience in good shape.

6. It motivates you from the inside.

7. Mental flexibility is also good for your body.

8. It allows you to bend, so you don't break.

'Vulnerability is a weakness'

As children we are vulnerable. If we are damaged around our vulnerability during childhood through simply not being taught enough helpful ways to look after ourselves (boundaries) or through more overt abuse and bullying, we grow into our adult bodies and are expected to be able to take care of ourselves. But the injured parts of our minds stay childlike and have to find ways of coping.

Your vulnerabilities are directly connected to your feelings. They tell you exactly where your work is. You'll know when you are in your vulnerability – it feels genuinely raw and exposing. Yet, it is not weakness; the feelings you are connecting with provide the information about the movements you need to feel safer and happier inside yourself. Working with vulnerability ultimately reduces stress reactions and emotional regressions and leaves you feeling calmer overall. Therefore, vulnerability is indeed a strength, not a weakness.

You can come back to these warm-up sections whenever you need to. In particular, if at any point you feel you are having difficulty connecting with the weekly and daily workouts, you might find it helpful to reactivate your core stability and range of motion to ensure your foundations are still strong.

Lastly, before we move on, cast your mind back to your

mental health goals. You might have a better idea now of how to set yourself up for them internally. Has anything come out of these warm-up exercises that you could use? For example, if one of your goals is to strengthen your self-esteem, making time for estimable actions and thoughts would be a good set-up. Or, if one of your goals is to work on your boundaries, making time to be around people with whom you feel safe to practise would set you up for a better chance of success.

As we move into the weekly and daily workouts, there will be lots of opportunities to both understand and action these more tangibly. For now, however, consider yourself warmed up and ready to go with the eight main workouts.

Chapter 4

YOUR WEEKLY MENTAL HEALTH WORKOUTS

IN THIS SECTION of the programme, you will find your weekly mental health workouts. Designed to ensure maximum opportunity for change and reduce your risk of psychological injury right now and going forward, they are also a really easy way to introduce structure into your week, which is fundamental to a healthy and happy mind.

Remember, extra planners and checklists are downloadable from www.yourmentalhealthworkout.com and you are welcome to use your separate journal to continue with the questions posed throughout.

Weekly Workouts Explained

Your weekly mental health workout programme looks like this:

1 x Therapeutic Space – the equivalent of a personal trainer

2 x Social Events – your mental health form and technique check-in

3 x Exercise – cardiovascular or other physical exercise, done in a way that benefits your mind

4 x Self-care – the fuel and nutrition to keep Your Mental Health Workout alive and pumping

If these workouts are new to you, it can take some time to get them in place. There is no time pressure here – just do your best with what you've got and seek to expand your resources as and when you can. If you are already doing some of them, that's great news and this programme can help you to progress your journey.

The weekly workouts target structure, safety, confidence and accountability. They offer you opportunities to work closely with your core stability and range of motion. They actively move you towards a lifestyle that is happy and healthy and, over a sustained period of time, they create psychological choice and integrity.

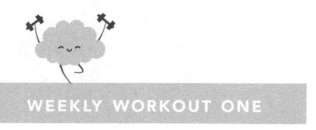

WEEKLY WORKOUT ONE

1 x Therapeutic Space

If this were a physical workout what is the first thing you would do?

You wouldn't just grab some weights and start pumping away. Ideally, you would look for guidance on how to start from someone who has the experience to help you identify and sustain your goals. Hopefully, they'd be someone you could trust and who has your best interests at heart.

In the context of a physical workout, that usually comes in the form of a personal trainer or group fitness teacher. For your mental health, it's a therapist, counsellor or a safe reflective space you can share with another person. Therapy can be found in many ways, and I have chosen to use the term 'therapeutic space' to loosen us up around the idea of what therapy looks like.

Having someone or somewhere that helps you to help yourself and checks in with you each week is where we shall start on Your Mental Health Workout journey.

In this workout, we will break down exactly what it means to 'have therapy', where to find it, how to find it and how to get the most out of it.

THERAPEUTIC SPACE WORKOUT

The workout itself is just three simple steps:

1. Decide what your preferred therapeutic space will look like.

2. Keep showing up.

3. Remain willing.

WHY WE DO THIS WORKOUT

For years, participating in a therapeutic space has been something we do when we are in emotional anguish and something is amiss. This belief has created a stigma and led to us feeling ashamed and secretive about doing for our minds what we do for our bodies without a second thought.

We do this workout because we live in a society where self-reliance is championed and yes, being able to support yourself is marvellous, but none of us gets it spot-on all the time. We all need someone or somewhere to depend on. It is proven that being allowed to depend on someone who can guide, teach and care for us fosters sustainable independence. Indeed, healthy dependence creates healthy independence.

We do this workout because yes, you could choose to lean

on family and friends for therapeutic support – in fact, your support system outside of therapy is a whole other workout (coming up next!). But having a therapeutic space is quite a different thing. It is much more objective and confidential than when you speak to family and friends. With them, we are prone to censoring ourselves because we feel embarrassed, angry with them or, sometimes, we want to protect them from something. Moreover, they are often what we want to talk about in therapy – so we do this workout to provide you with an objective, confidential and dependable space to talk about yourself and your life and explore your feelings.

Having said that, therapy isn't just talking about your feelings. It involves an educated plan, dedicated consistency and an approach that family and friends cannot provide. It is often the place where you start to experiment with your newly activated core stability and explore your range of motion and psychological edges in the hands of people who know exactly what to do, or have the support network to help them work on their own boundaries and vulnerability so that you do not have to worry, as much, about the consequences of changing your behaviour in their presence.

Lastly, we do this workout because we all have emotional pain, although you do not have to be 'unwell' or even psychologically out of shape to do it. You don't go to the gym because you are broken. In fact, you *can't* go if you are broken. You go because you want to be fitter, stronger and happier. And we do this workout to give our minds the same privilege.

HOW TO GET THIS WORKOUT WORKING FOR YOU

There are a number of options to get what is known as 'therapy' working for you. You do not have to be sitting in front of someone, baring your soul, if that doesn't appeal.

As with going to the gym and training your body, some people prefer to work out in isolation and others love group exercise classes, and your mind has similar options. The important thing to remember is that your therapy can be as private as you want it to be. We live in an age where we are encouraged to self-promote and share parts of our lives that have never been on show before, yet privacy is important to all of us to different extents.

It is important to remember that just like personal trainers, therapeutic spaces are not magic: you are going to have to put in the hard work in the same way you would if you were working on your body. Your therapeutic space is unlikely to offer advice, but they will offer helpful observations, pose questions you may not have thought about before and support you to develop all the skills we are learning in this programme. If this was a physical workout, you wouldn't become fitter or stronger just by attending a class; you'd get fitter and stronger by working hard during the class. And that, in the main, is how you get this workout working for you.

Part of my mission is to make a defined therapeutic space feel as normal to you as having any other healthcare professional in your life – doctor, physio, nutritionist, you name it.

There is one major difference here between the psychological and physical workouts. Within your mental health workouts it is the afterburn of your therapeutic space, the things you take forward into your life, that really create change. In contrast to your physical workouts where change is created when you are in direct contact with your personal trainer or in your class, your personal therapeutic bests will happen outside of your therapeutic space.

FINDING A THERAPEUTIC SPACE THAT WORKS FOR YOU

One of the hardest parts of this programme will be identifying the kind of therapeutic space you'd like. There are counsellors, therapists, psychotherapists, psychologists, recovery groups, support groups, peer-support groups . . . And within all of these are different approaches and skill sets to pick from. So keep this in mind: ultimately, this workout is about *your* relationship with your therapeutic space and how *you* use it; your personal trainer will help support you, but you have to put in the hard work.

Any space where you have the input of a trained and more experienced other, an opportunity to reflect with those on a similar journey or simply feel safe enough to be honest with yourself, counts as your therapy workout. If you have chosen do Your Mental Health Workout in a pair or a group, you might consider meeting up each week to share your experience and reflect alongside each other.

You must feel able to speak about yourself without the interruption of others' opinions, advice or experiences. Preferably, this is in the company of at least one other person; however, if you are adamant that you'd rather do this alone, you can create time in your week for self-reflection as a modification; but please be aware that – in this context – self-reflection is not therapy.

Ask yourself:

- What results would you like to achieve by having a therapeutic space?
- Do you want to work with a male, female or gender-neutral therapist?
- Does your therapeutic space need a specific focus – say, anxiety? Addiction? Bulimia? Grief?
- Where in your weekly programme can you fit it in – i.e. which day and time? (Most therapeutic spaces happen at the same time each week.)
- Can you fund it? How will you fund it? Do you have a budget available? Do you use health insurance? Would you prefer something that doesn't cost much?
- How long do you want to be in therapy? Just the five weeks of this programme or do you see yourself introducing it as a fixture in your life? (This may change over the coming weeks, but it's interesting to know where you are at right now.)

If you choose to see a therapist, counsellor, psychologist or other mental health professional, here are the basics to look out for:

Warmth and compassion
Your therapist should give you the feeling that things can be done with kindness and compassion. This doesn't mean that they'll put up with unreasonable behaviours or attitudes. They should be able to maintain reasonable warmth while holding psychological and physical boundaries, and

also be comfortable challenging you when appropriate and necessary.

Acceptance

In therapy you should feel accepted for who you are. You should have the psychological space to open up and, over time, to let your defences down.

Accountability

The accountability of showing up to therapy is yours, but in many ways in the therapeutic space both you and your mental health professional are accountable. Accountability means engaging with all the parts of you that create your present moment. When you do this workout – when you show up – you are accountable. You are nurturing a basic human dependency need, and training yourself to remain committed and consistent.

Vulnerability

We talked a lot about vulnerability in the warm-up (see pp. 47–64) and in terms of your therapeutic space, it's important to remember that the power of vulnerability is stronger than most of us expect. It can be subtle, but it is mighty. If you are able to be authentically vulnerable and accepting of it in your therapeutic space, you have access to be empowered through love and compassion. Love and compassion are psychological drives that are far more nurturing and effective than any motivation that comes out of shame and self-loathing.

73

Congruence

In terms of your therapeutic space workout, you are looking for a place where you can hold yourself in an honest and harmonious way. Being congruent means that your behaviour matches how you feel; it is the opposite of cognitive dissonance (see p. 19). The atmosphere in your therapeutic space needs to be consistent, loving, connective and containing.

Once you have identified your chosen therapeutic space, be it psychotherapy, group support, peer support, etc. (see p. 231 for some suggestions of therapeutic spaces that might work for you), this workout is quite simple.

HOW TO SHOW UP FOR THIS WORKOUT

In the warm-up exercises on pp. 36 and 48, we looked extensively at your core stability and range of motion. Your therapeutic space is an immediate opportunity to practise these. If you choose an individual session, you'll have the undivided attention of a professional to help you practise at a pace the suits you. If you go down the group route you can (ideally) trust that the people around you are also working on similar stuff and have their own support systems in place; this should make it safe for you to practise new things. Show up in as many ways as possible: physically be on time, emotionally show up by working with your feelings in real time and, most importantly, show up for yourself by being as honest as you feel able to be.

While doing this workout, there will be sessions in which nothing much happens. Do not be disheartened, you have still completed step 2 of the workout. Just by showing up you give yourself the message that you care, and you believe you are worth it; this is, in fact, one of the best stabilising movements you can do for your core stability. So just stick to the plan, even if you don't really want to be there on any given day.

Tip: remember, this is five weeks to a healthier mind, so give it five weeks before you make a decision about whether you'd like to introduce regular therapy into your weekly routine as a lifestyle choice.

The serious bit: red flags in therapy

Clearly, I am an advocate of weekly therapy sessions. Which means I also need to talk to you about the things that can go wrong.

Most mental health professionals are trained to be as neutral as possible. They are also human beings with minds just like yours, however, and not all therapeutic relationships work out.

Anyone holding therapeutic spaces should be abiding by the ethics of their governing body (in the UK examples are BACP, FDAP and UKCP). You should easily be able to find out which governing body your therapeutic space is regulated by and what their ethical guidelines are. If you notice something that seems unethical, you can raise it – first with the person in question and then with the governing body itself. If individual therapists or counsellors do not appear to be registered with a relevant governing body, I suggest you do not consult them.

Support groups are slightly different but should still have ethical guidelines that they abide by. Ideally, you should be able to find these on their website.

Some therapists share more of themselves than others and you might get to know a little bit about where your therapist comes from. Ultimately, however, you ought to be the main focus in your therapeutic relationship. Social invitations and any kind of sexual misconduct – whether physical or verbal – is considered unethical.

The great thing about this workout (and most of the workouts in this programme) is that you cannot get it wrong. You can make it harder for yourself through being dishonest about your thoughts, feelings and behaviours – just like working with a personal trainer and not applying their recommendations, or having cheat days – but you cannot get it wrong. Please remind yourself of this and if you find yourself thinking that you are getting something 'wrong', please share these thoughts in your therapeutic space, so you can counteract that unhelpful internal chatter from the get-go.

Now, some of you out there will still be scrunching up your noses and telling yourselves that you're not sure you have time for therapy in your week (although many are now available online, meaning less of a time investment), that it won't work for you, that someone else probably needs it more than you or you don't want to spend your hard-earned money on it. We call this ambivalence, and most therapists are very skilled at working with it. A decent one will work with you in whatever shape you arrive in, good, bad or ugly, as long as it is within their skill set. They may also be able to make recommendations for further or different support if they think it would benefit you more. And, as above, if you are absolutely not ready for this, then self-reflection is a good modification for you to start with.

Funding your therapeutic space

If you cannot afford to pay for therapy, try one of the free or low-cost therapeutic spaces listed on p. 232. I have led with the therapeutic space workout because it is something we can do just once a week (rather than two or three times), and while it may seem pivotal, please do not panic about it or indeed dismiss it; keep in mind that working a programme like Your Mental Health Workout is developing a therapeutic-space inside of you too, and if your therapeutic space workout needs to be added in at a later date due to financial or time constraints, that is perfectly OK.

YOUR THERAPEUTIC SPACE: POINTS TO KEEP IN MIND

1. **The actual work done within the therapeutic space is about helping you to look after yourself.** Depending on the approach of the therapist, this will vary. I like to focus on the different parts of you: the healthy part, the young part, the shy part, the happy part, the sad part, the shamed part, the destructive part and so on. I find the separating out of 'parts' and reintegrating them helpful; if therapy were a

physical workout, this would be the equivalent of leg day, upper body day, chest day, etc. Therapy allows you to assess how each section of you is functioning and if anything hurts, hinders or simply needs tweaking. In each session, you get to dismantle metaphorically, with kindness and compassion, any equipment you might have been using ineffectively – likely because no one has showed you how to use it properly, until now. You get to look at unhelpful habits that might get in the way of you realising your potential, find new options and fresh prospects for transformation. Your therapist will be able to spot the things that cause you pain and the discrepancies within you that you consciously or unconsciously avoid. They will help you come to understand where those contradictions come from and why they are likely to contribute to an experience of pain, tension, conflict and disturbance. All in aid of helping you look after the integrity of your mind.

2. Therapy is a reparative relationship. Those of you who have experienced relational trauma and any other type of disturbance in your life will know, sense or feel that there are yearnings and unmet needs within you. Therapy is the place where you learn to meet these needs within yourself and how to effectively ask others to meet your needs too by practising in the relationship with your therapeutic space. By watching how your therapist, group or peers do it for you first, you can often heal wounds and ruptures you didn't even know you had. Therapeutic spaces allow you to borrow some of their wellness, hope, pride and health until you are able to get your own. I am a strong believer that we need external love, validation and attention so that we can learn how to give it to ourselves. How can you be expected to be loving, gentle and compassionate towards yourself if you haven't been shown how to do it? Therapeutic spaces offer an opportunity not found anywhere else.

3. All sorts of things happen in therapy. You're likely to laugh and cry during the process. You'll discover your personal irony and contradictions, make mistakes in a safe atmosphere and gift yourself the freedom of choice about how you use your mental health muscle going forward. Everything that happens in your therapy workout is part of your healing, it's all part of discovering what balance and wellness feel like to you.

4. Everyone is entitled to therapy. This is for those of you whose core stability is not quite where we need it right now and who are struggling to justify the time, effort and investment a therapeutic space requires. Maybe you think there is someone else out there who has it worse and your mind tells you they deserve a spot in therapy instead of you. Please do not sideline your pain for people and situations you don't even know: someone else's broken leg does not mean that your sprained ankle doesn't need attention. You deserve a seat in therapy as much as anyone else, purely because you want it and are willing to do the work. I bet you have never questioned whether you 'deserve' to go to the gym or 'are worth' a physical workout! Don't compare your suffering to someone else's. Just the fact that you want to be in the therapy chair means you are entitled to be there.

A WORD ON COST

It is common knowledge that some therapy can be pricey. What may not be so well known is what exactly you are paying for when you commit to attending a therapeutic space.

As well as paying for your hour (or more), your fee is paying for that person's attention on your body language, your verbal communication, your thoughts, your feelings, your process. It also pays for the planning, thinking and feeling that goes into your treatment outside of sessions about what's going be helpful for you. And it covers the cost, in part, for your therapist to be supervised, so they and you can be sure they are doing their very best for you, or at the very least that no harm is being done. A supervision also ensures that they are fit to practise – i.e. that their own mental health is in good shape. Some of it also goes towards your therapist's therapy. Yep, therapists need therapists too; mine is pretty black belt, I have to say. It is so important for us to know what it feels like to be in the client's position, feeling vulnerable, resistant, challenged, scared and accountable.

So even though you see your therapeutic space for just an hour or two a week (in fact, the therapeutic hour is usually fifty minutes), there is a lot more involved that ensures the space is truly secure, confidential, helpful, safe, contained and moderated for you.

Your therapeutic space is an investment in you and a good experience will stay with you for life. That is why therapy comes first in our weekly mental health workouts – it gives us the external support we all need in life and makes us feel able to challenge ourselves throughout the rest of the workout.

YOUR MENTAL HEALTH WORKOUT WEEKLY CHECKLIST

WEEKLY WORKOUTS	M	T	W	TH	F	S	SU
THERAPY							
SOCIAL EVENTS							
EXERCISE							
SELF-CARE							

DAILY WORKOUTS							
MINDFULNESS							
CONNECTION							
APPRECIATION							
MOVEMENT							

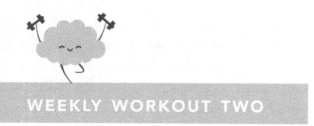

2 x Social Events

Because mental health is something that we can't see, even the most consistent of us might not be able to visualise and tangibly understand the changes that take place as we sit in our therapeutic space or work on our mental health alone. How do we check on this stuff when we are working on our bodies? Well, we tend to look in the mirror or at what other people are doing . . .

You might already be aware of how important socialising is in helping you to heal and take good care of your mental health. There is so much information stored in our relationships with others that without them it is very difficult to practise and process everything we covered in the warm-up and all that you will be (or have already been) working on in your therapeutic space.

Using your new-found stability and range of motion within your social life helps you to make informed changes going forward and contributes to finding a healthy balance between alone time and socialising events. As part of Your Mental Health Workout, social events are primarily representative of your form and technique check-in. They also help you to assess and satisfy your social-arousal levels, which are equivalent to you determining how intense a workout you'd like to have on any given day. They can also act as a diagnostic tool and a great reference point for how you are doing with the rest of your workout – and, of course, heal any injuries stemming from old, unhelpful social habits.

So . . . let's get you moving.

SOCIAL EVENTS WORKOUT

STEP 1: Social arousal levels

In the first instance, use the information in this chapter to assess your current desire to socialise and compare it to what is usual for you. I am asking you simply to become aware of any changes in your personal desire to socialise.

Note: at this point, this is just about listing things you would like to do – no action is necessary right now if you are not up to it.

List four social events (here or in your journal) that you would like to include in the weeks ahead:

1.

2.

3.

4.

Pick two that seem likely to satisfy your social needs, based on your observations of yourself today. You can then make contact with people who might be able to socialise with you in this way, and write your action plans on your planner.

STEP 2: Form and technique check-in

When you feel ready, action the items from the list above and use your social events as an opportunity to get some mirroring and reflection while with others or in hindsight. Ask yourself:

- What do/did you notice about your core stability and your range of motion?
- What happens/happened in your thoughts and feelings?

STEP 3: Diagnostic information

Much of the information gathered in the above two steps can inform what you need to work on and any injuries that need attending to. For example, if you notice that each time you are with a particular person your core stability is challenged or you can't hold your boundaries when someone seems angry or hurt, these are opportunities for you to practise your mental health workouts in real time.

STEP 4: Healing

You know when you are healing physically it can sometimes feel quite painful, itchy and frustrating? Well, when you are healing relational injuries within your psychology, the same thing happens. Notice your thoughts, feelings and behaviours, your equipment, your mental health muscle responses and the results you get . . . The healing happens when you stop judging and comparing and start using this information for change. For example, if each time you are with a particular person or group of people you find yourself comparing yourself to them, your social events challenge is to stop comparing and understand that we are all equal as human beings. It won't feel comfortable, but repetition supports you in managing your anxiety to feel more confident and happy. You could start with this example or create one of your own.

WHY WE DO THIS WORKOUT
We do this workout because we are social creatures. We need to be socialised regularly or else our mental health suffers. This is connected to our attachment styles and experiences of both peers and authority figures throughout our lives. We will delve further into this when we look at the connection workout (see p. 149), but for now I want you to understand why regular social interaction motivates, inspires and helps you to learn and grow.

We are hardwired for progression, learning and connection. We are supposed to be pack animals; therefore, if the opportunity to be part of a pack does not present itself or we are isolating or avoiding social situations due to social anxiety, depression, a pandemic, cultural shame, shame in general or fear, we become naturally exhausted by the internal effort of trying to keep our feelings, thoughts and behaviours balanced. And when we repress our emotions, anxiety and depression thrive.

Furthermore, when we are social, we aim to belong, to feel seen, witnessed and understood; we are better able to process things and create healthy progressions for ourselves. We make ourselves available to be supported and kindly challenged, therefore we get an improved felt sense of the equilibrium our minds pursue. So we do this workout because we all have heaps of feelings about the things that happen in our social lives and it is an opportunity to practise working with these in real time.

If our social needs do not get met, psychological distress and injury are more likely to emerge. Distress shows up in all sorts of shapes and sizes, and changes in how we are internally and externally in social events are usually the first indication that something is not quite right, which is why I asked you to assess your current desire to socialise and compare it to what is 'normal' for you. Anything from cancelling social engagements and spending too much time alone to being overly social and not spending any time alone (or any changes in between) is an indication of something worth paying attention to within your mental health.

And we do this workout to heal our hearts. Whether you are prone to over- or under- socialising, it is most likely that you have been hurt, at some point, by something that has happened socially, and the injuries you have from being in relationships heal in relationships.

HOW TO GET THIS WORKOUT WORKING FOR YOU

Getting this workout working for you is all about knowing what your social needs actually are and taking responsibility to get them met.

We are aiming for balance, always: sufficient socialising that you can use to energise, adjust and correct yourself, but not so much that you end up comparing yourself to others and developing unhelpful judgments. Please remember that this is, in part, a diagnostic workout that simply informs you of what you might like to change. It is not a comparative exercise.

When we do physical workouts, for the first few minutes our brain releases chemicals that can make us feel as if we are threatened, and it takes a while for our minds and bodies to realise what's happening and sync with each other. A similar thing happens when we enter social situations, which is why, when I work on this stuff in therapy with clients, I usually negotiate some kind of rule in order to get it working for them, such as: 'Exercise or work is not allowed to take priority over social events'; or, 'Go to the event and if you are still unhappy about being there, you can leave after thirty minutes'. If we are prone to isolation, we often need some kind of prod to get us there and then our brain chemistry takes over and things start to feel a bit better. In the opposite direction, the rules we come up with might be something like, 'Set a required maximum on the number of social engagements in a week' or, 'Stick to two social events' in order to allow space to do the rest of Your Mental Health Workout'.

FIGURING OUT YOUR SOCIAL-AROUSAL LEVELS
(INTENSITY LEVELS)

As above, for some of you two social events per week might feel like a lot and for others not enough. That will depend on your personality, **which does not need changing**, just being sensitised to, so we can make sure this workout is effective for you. When you go to the gym, you are not trying to change the fundamentals of your body, but simply to fine-tune what you've already got and find a way to feel good about it. Likewise, you may already have a good handle on your social needs – maybe you know that you have to have your own space or that being with others is optimal for you – but if not, the easiest way to estimate them is to ask your-self: do you recharge alone or with others?

If you recharge alone, regardless of your other personality traits, you are classified as an introvert. If you recharge around other people, again regardless of how outgoing you are, you fall into the extrovert category. These categories have no further bearing on how shy or confident you might be, nor are they predictors of your mental wellbeing. It is also unlikely that you are a pure introvert or a pure extrovert – a bit like our bodies, our minds generally prefer one thing, but every now and again, depending on circumstances, they benefit from a bit of variation.

You can be introverted, quiet in social situations and have a preference for being alone, while being quite self-assured and confident, with your self-esteem in good shape. Introverts are not necessarily shy people. Shyness is a family member of shame, so being shy is quite a painful place to be, while being introverted can be quite comfortable. Take my story from the start of the book as an example (see p. xi) – that painfully shy experience I had was indeed indicative of my mental health, my social anxiety, and I was able to work through it over a number of years, with the right people around me. I would now classify myself firmly as a confident introvert. I can spend a lot of time alone and I recharge alone and because I allow space for this, I am able to be confident, outgoing and socialise often.

MENTAL HEALTH MYTH

*'Introverts don't like to be around people
and they are scared of people; extroverts want
attention and talk too much'*

TRUTH: Introverts just don't like to be around people for as long as someone who is extroverted, they are not scared they just need a good enough reason to interact with others, they tend not to speak up just for the sake of it, they process their thoughts in silence. They find small talk difficult but love to chat about something they have an interest in. They often have a few very close friends whom they value highly and can be intimate with. Introverts need people whom they can respect and trust and who will stay in their lives for a long while.

Meanwhile, extroverts may appear like they want to pull attention and speak aloud a lot more often; all this is just a processing style. Extroverts are not just talking to take up space, they are trying to figure something out. To the introvert this might appear like pointless talking but to the extrovert this is a vital attempt to understand a situation or a decision. Remember the extrovert is not as confident as they might appear – they also experience self-doubt but at the same time are more able to cope with high levels of social stimuli.

If you are extroverted, you may appear outgoing and confident because you like to be around others a lot of the time and therefore look like you've got it all together, but you might also need a lot of support and find yourself frustrated when others assume you are the 'strong' one. The assumptions that people make about extroverts can be quite inaccurate and often leave them feeling unseen and misunderstood around their social needs.

There is also a middle ground: the ambivert. If you find that your social needs vary from day to day, week to week, you might be an ambivert. For ambiverts, the process is much more trial and error. You will need to check in with yourself to see where your social arousal level is and what would be the most helpful execution of this particular mental health workout on a day-to-day basis. Over these five weeks, you might start spotting patterns. For example, maybe you'll notice that at the start of the week, you get your energy from being around people, whereas towards the end, you feel more refreshed from being alone. Your pattern might show up on a daily, weekly or monthly cycle. Make a note of it on your planner so you can tailor this workout to you.

Which category do you see yourself in?

Now go back to the workout on p. 85 and make your social event plans.

A word on social anxiety

Although anxiety is woven in and out of the programme, it seems particularly apt in this chapter to give social anxiety a specific focus, since those who experience it might feel quite challenged and find this workout a little more painful than others, and I want to make space for that.

I talk about anxiety often throughout this book as something that happens in response to our minds becoming overloaded and unable to process what is happening. Our feelings are then repressed and, as a result, we have a physiological response that we call anxiety.

Give yourself the space and time to practise letting yourself be supported and feel seen and witnessed in your therapeutic environment by talking about the anxieties you experience related to social events. Whether you are a socially anxious introvert, extrovert or ambivert, you will need to have some self-soothing behaviours for going into social events, such as positive and helpful self-talk and an option to leave if it gets too much (but don't use the latter as a cop-out, please). Then, as the muscle strengthens and stretches and your technique improves (and you feel confident to do so), you can start to include this workout in your weekly plan. You might also like to take a visit to the physio section, where you can get a targeted approach to social anxiety (see p. 219).

Finding balance can be quite tricky when other people are involved, but over time, as you do more form and technique check-ins with yourself via this social events workout, you'll be able to judge when to increase or decrease the number of social events you include. Considering many of us have busy lives I suggest keeping your baseline at two per week for the five weeks of Your Mental Health Workout and within this you can increase or decrease the number of people involved or the time spent at each event. You could also find balance through choosing activities such as eating out, cooking with someone, exercising, shopping or going for a walk – things that allow you to interact with other people in a way you find relaxing and soothing (a sign that your nervous system is happy and balanced).

YOUR MENTAL HEALTH WORKOUT WEEKLY CHECKLIST

WEEKLY WORKOUTS	M	T	W	TH	F	S	SU
THERAPY							
SOCIAL EVENTS							
EXERCISE							
SELF-CARE							

DAILY WORKOUTS							
MINDFULNESS							
CONNECTION							
APPRECIATION							
MOVEMENT							

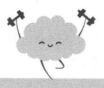

3 x Exercise

So far, we have concentrated exclusively on your mind, and trying to help you find ways of making it happier and healthier. Historically, for the sake of ease within the health and wellbeing industry, we have habitually separated body and mind, and it is this separation that has allowed us to neglect our mental health in favour of physical health. However, your third weekly mental health workout is where we help to align you in both body and mind.

For the purpose of this programme, I have added physical exercise here as a distinct mental health workout because, with a little tweaking, your three weekly workout sessions can be made to work twice as hard, developing your inner resilience as well as your physical strength.

For some people, going to the gym is therapy in itself, and I want to advance the therapeutic and healing benefits of exercise here by giving you some mental health workouts to apply during physical exercise, if you so wish. But please know that exercise, done with love, will always be helpful to your mental health.

Your Mental Health Workout is designed with a baseline

of **3 x 30 minutes' exercise per week**. Depending on your physical and emotional needs, you could take this up to five times per week. Or, if at any point you feel unable to physically work out because you are tired, injured etc., I totally support you in practising good self-care (see Weekly Workout Four, p. 115) around exercise and making your physical workout as light as possible or necessary.

EXERCISE WORKOUT

Take your physical workout to the next level by specifically and intentionally targeting your mental health at the same time.

1. **Monitor how you feel about exercising, while exercising.** So often we go into our workouts mindlessly. Let's start to concentrate on engaging the body and mind simultaneously. Over time, you can actively overlap your mindfulness workout here (see p. 134) as an optional progression to enhance your experience.

2. **Get even more specific. Check in with your thoughts and feelings about your body.** What is your self-talk doing? Exercise is a great time to start to change any negative self-talk that pops up. We will expand on this in the daily workouts (see pp. 131–189). As a progression, over time, you can also apply your appreciation workout (see p. 170) while you are physically exercising to get the best for your mind.

3. **Notice what happens to your mental health muscle if you skip a physical workout.** What feelings do you have? Do you give yourself a hard time? Can you work with those awkward feelings and use the opportunity to strengthen your mental health muscle, rather than

using them to bully yourself into doing unwanted physical exercise?

4. What do the feelings you find tell you? What is your call to action?

WHY WE DO THIS WORKOUT

Exercise without any additional psychological work behind it is already well known as an effective way to help manage mood and mental health. Research points to relief from symptoms of anxiety, depression, stress and trauma. Exercise has also shown up as an effective way to develop self-esteem, boundaries and, of course, your actual physical core stability and range of motion. Based on this research, it seems clear why we do this workout.

We are also aligning mental with physical health here, rather than viewing any mental health benefits as a useful by-product. And of course, this is where this whole metaphor started! There I was going from the therapy room to the gym, and over time, I couldn't help but notice the parallels. In many ways, the gains were similar if not identical to each other.

In the three years leading up to writing this programme I was inspired by the London fitness industry and developed a fascination with what happens in our brains during physical exercise that makes it feel so helpful? I found thousands of studies on the positive changes to our minds observed post exercise, but what I really wanted to know was what was happening there *during* exercise. Yes, we know the basics: the hippocampus swells and the amygdala can be activated (these are parts of the brain) – but what does that mean for a therapeutic or healing journey?

I have been lucky enough to consult on mental health for a number of gyms, so have had ample time to observe and gather information about this exact question. Through already well-known research coupled with studies of myself, my clients and my peers and asking the same questions I have posed to you above, I have observed that a regular exercise routine mixed with a mental health workout provides immense therapeutic benefit.

But how?

The biochemical response in the mind when exercising allows you to enter a psychological state where you have access to feelings and thoughts you might usually remain less conscious of or just choose to avoid.

In part, the reason exercise is so helpful is because usually when we have a feeling or a thought that we don't understand it makes us anxious and we'd rather not deal with it. The mind and body come up with ways to discharge that energy and our primal compulsions take control. When exercising, however, our energy is focused on the task in hand and there is much less risk that behavioural impulses or compulsions will overtake (the exception being if we are in the grasp of an addiction). During physical exercise the mind might feel less defended. This is because, when exercising, we are using our bodies to look after ourselves, rather than relying exclusively on our minds. So, as the mind and body start working together (usually about ten minutes into a physical workout), the mind can start to feel safer – and when we feel safe and protected, there is no need for our defences to activate. This provides the internal psychological movements we need to process difficult mind and body experiences. Take conflict, for example: many of us (but not all) find conflict a difficult thing to process because we are frightened of potential, perceived or real rejection and anger. If you've ever physically worked out following a difficult event or conversation, you'll probably have experienced a sense of clarity and relief afterwards that allows you to better cope with, approach and assimilate new information.

Modern exercise trends appear to be aware of this and use it to advantage. We see large groups of people in workout communities celebrating everyone who walks through the door for showing up, for working hard, for trying new things . . . very similar to what happens in a therapeutic space. People are affirmed for personal milestones and community interaction. Some fitness companies have even developed the technology to allow us to access this experience in our own homes. They also use all sorts of positive messaging, and I have worked with brands that want to specifically programme therapeutic intervention into their workouts. I am sure that the next level of fitness will include our minds.

A LITTLE BIT OF SCIENCE

If you have ever been in a distressing situation and found yourself calm and collected, despite the circumstances, it is because your mind has very skilfully released endorphins – the 'feel-good' hormone produced in the mind, by the mind to block out physical and emotional pain – essentially numbing you. When we exercise, we have a comparable experience, so we tend to feel less emotional pain too. Endorphins are effective because they allow you to survive psychologically or physically threatening situations. During exercise they help you to challenge yourself and take yourself to your physical edges, and knowing what we know now, we can also use this opportunity to confront the lesser-known areas of our minds.

With an endorphin hit you might experience a feeling of happiness kicking in during or after your workout. You might already know about serotonin; it is the mood-boosting neurotransmitter. Unlike endorphins, which block pain and boost pleasure, serotonin promotes pleasure itself. In fact, the most commonly prescribed antidepressant is an SSRI (selective serotonin reuptake inhibitor). SSRIs work by increasing serotonin levels in your brain via demobilising the reuptake process, as their name suggests, so that the neurotransmitter hangs around for longer. Serotonin is released when you exercise and is the chemical that allows you to change mood, perspective and generally feel happier post-workout. It has been said that exercise is the most underused antidepressant.

The other thing that might be of interest to you is that when you exercise, a protein called BDNF (brain-derived neurotropic factor) is active. BDNF promotes cognitive health, memory and the way you learn and ensures the survival and growth of the neurones themselves. BDNF also maintains effective transmission of chemical messages between brain cells and is vital for your mental health. When participating in any mental health workout you need this protein to uphold positive changes in your mind as it sustains new, healthy neuropathways. If we were to wrap some kind of muscle support around your mind to help you function, this would be it.

Exercise can change the brain in ways that talking therapy cannot because of the swelling in the hippocampus, which is the part of your mind that is heavily involved with learning, long-term memory and emotional responses. It works closely with the amygdala, which is where any trauma or chronic stress are stored; in this part of the mind, we are effectively programmed by our genetics and our life experiences; this is where unconscious trauma lives. When you exercise your brain pathways, neurotransmitters and less conscious processes are wide open to taking in new information, making potential changes and receiving the effects of talking therapy in a much more efficient and effective way. This also means you can target an extremely unique and sensitive human experience if you choose to make your physical workout a mental health workout as well.

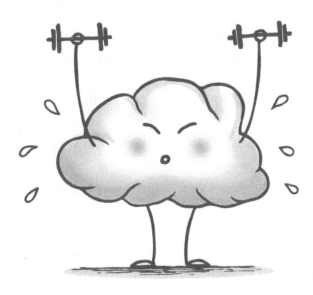

HOW TO GET THIS WORKOUT WORKING FOR YOU

Knowing what you know now, it is probably easier to understand why exercise is one of the most natural and effective self-regulation tools for your mental health. In fact, all of Your Mental Health Workout contributes to managing stress.

Stress is a simple physiological reaction involving your brain, your immune system and, eventually, your nervous system. When you describe yourself as stressed, you are probably talking about a sense of tension, but it is important to understand that the tension is not actually what defines stress; rather, it is a symptom. Using exercise to manage the symptom is very helpful, but if you really want to get physical exercise working well for your mental health, you have to get underneath that and make this workout effective by applying the therapeutic tools and questions at the start of this chapter.

We need stress to help us protect our safety and survival. Stress is the mental health equivalent to what physical pain does in a physical workout. If you developed shooting pains in your knee while running, hopefully you'd take that as a sign to stop running until it is better and it is safe for your knee to be back in action. If you develop symptoms of stress in your mind, you also need to stop and give yourself a chance to feel safe psychologically once more. Yet, sometimes we don't get the message that we are safe again and we remain in a stressed response. Getting this workout working for you means understanding your personal stress responses and responding with the appropriate type of physical exercise. (See also 'Stress', p.210.)

WHAT TYPE OF EXERCISE IS RIGHT FOR YOUR MENTAL HEALTH?

Each and every body is made for a slightly different way of moving, as is every mind. When we bring them together to manage stress, as well as some of your other feelings, we have to ensure you are getting the best out of both worlds.

Here are some things to consider when deciding the type of physical workout that would work best for you and your mind.

Weightlifting

Weightlifting and strength training are effective forms of exercise if you find that your main source of stress is in your thoughts, whether short-lived, long-lived or intrusive (see pp. 9–10). You will probably also have trouble making decisions, reality checking and problem solving. You will most likely also find that you have difficulty setting boundaries, visible and invisible (see pp. 54–5), and using your psychological strength effectively. When we strengthen our bodies, we feel physically stronger, and because body and mind want to feel aligned, the mind tends also to feel stronger and more able to protect itself.

Yoga, Pilates and Barre

These workouts are really effective for people whose psychological imbalances (stress) tend to be rooted in their feelings. If you sometimes feel full of feeling and a bit overwhelmed, but are unsure as to why, this is your best option. You need time and space to help integrate your thoughts and feelings, so you can process and understand what your mind and body are trying to tell you. Lower-intensity workouts where you can keep control of your breath and use the movement as a moving meditation are going to be beneficial for you.

High-intensity Interval Training (HIIT)

This is great for using up excess cortisol and adrenaline that build up in our nervous systems. However, HIIT can also activate cortisol and, therefore, a trauma reaction in your mind: the fight-flight-freeze response. During a HIIT workout your cortisol levels spike and hopefully then drop after the workout to a lower level than before you started. This can be helpful because it forces your mind to find ways to manage that spike and, provided you do not remain in the trauma reaction (that your cortisol does indeed drop) after the workout, it teaches your mind that you are more capable of tolerating intensity than you might think. If you have ever struggled with addictions or disordered eating when you are stressed, HIIT workouts can help to avoid the acting-out stage, but you must use them to process what is going on in your mind, rather than purge and discharge it, otherwise you just replace the acting out with exercise, which can become a problem in itself.

Aerobic exercise

Swimming, cycling, walking, rowing and running are really good for the part of your mind that stores trauma, memories and unconscious emotions. This type of exercise allows the mind to open up in a way that we usually defend against in our day-to-day lives. I myself have had many an experience where I haven't quite been able to connect with why I feel angry, sad, excited, until it all falls into place while cycling home or going for a run. The hippocampus (see p. 104) opens up during aerobic exercise, and it is my belief that many people who enjoy this type of workout are unconsciously attempting to heal from trauma.

A word of caution

Just a little warning: gyms can be breeding grounds for unhelpful competition and comparisons. When doing exercise as part of Your Mental Health Workout, do it out of love for and connection with your body, rather than as a punishment. Punishing, comparing and judging yourself only plunge you into shame and self-loathing, making exercise a chore that will only hinder your mental health. The result, ultimately, being that it will be unlikely that you will be able to sustain a lifestyle that includes a healthy relationship with exercise.

If you find going to a gym particularly triggering, there is always the option of joining 'at- home' programmes. The motivation might be more difficult, but if this is the best option for your mind, then please do take it. You can also use the daily movement workout (see p. 184) if this type of exercise is just not good for you right now.

'You have to find a way to enjoy exercise'

Well, yes, it *is* helpful if you find a way to exercise that you enjoy, *but not everyone enjoys it, and you don't have to.* The important thing is that not enjoying exercise should not mean you don't do it. Your mind and body still need it to stay healthy, and exercise is likely to help balance your mood and reduce stress overall, regardless of how much gratification you get out of it. If you just don't like exercise and don't think you ever will, it is likely that you have some underlying core beliefs about it and what it means. For example, do you default to: 'Exercise means I am trying to change my body shape or weight'? Or, 'Only happy people exercise'? Or maybe it's a self-worth issue: 'I don't deserve/ feel good enough about my body to exercise'? My suggestion is that you pay attention to any core beliefs you hold in relationship to physical exercise and use the core-stability workout (see p. 36) to support you with finding a way to think about it in a way that is helpful to you.

If you see yourself in the examples above, consider your 3 x 30 minutes per week as something you are doing for the good of your mind, mood and wellbeing. It does not have to be about the shape of your body or overall fitness levels at all; make it about your mental health and see what happens.

EXERCISE AND EMOTIONS

Understood fully and used healthily, exercise can be a brilliant way to connect with your body and access and process the feelings you usually deny in other situations. For example, have you ever worked out angry? I am sure you'll have experienced the flush of extra strength you get when you are conscious of the emotion – the anger (in this case) literally acting as an energy enhancer. Ever done a yoga class with sadness bubbling under the surface and found you were able to release the tears during or after the class? If you exercise to flush out that extra charge and feel more able to cope afterwards, you are moving beyond the escapism that exercise can provide; plus, you give yourself an opportunity to work out your mental health muscle.

If you use exercise to rid yourself of uncomfortable emotions, ignoring your feelings as you go, however, you do yourself a disservice and forfeit the opportunity to strengthen your mental health muscle. Use exercise as a tool for processing emotion rather than discharging it, taking responsibility and being accountable for your mental health.

MENTAL HEALTH MYTH

'Physical tension is the main indicator of stress'

Just because you are not physically tense, that does not mean you are not stressed. Some of the most stressed people I have come across have an ability to appear physically calm. Stress shows up in many forms: disturbed sleep, changes in appetite, feeling irritable, trouble with making decisions, problems with remembering things . . . Well before our bodies feel the tension of stress, our minds are attempting to regulate us, and that means, when stressed, much of the mind's energy is being pumped into finding chemical balance. Because of this, the parts of the mind that are usually energised and available for making good decisions, remembering things and regulating sleep and appetite are effectively hijacked. The tension we eventually experience in the body is, in fact, chronic stress, and is an indication that we have been off balance for way too long. Sadly, we live in a society that seems to promote and facilitate living this way by affirming those who overwork, go 'above and beyond' and sacrifice themselves, but it is not good for our health. So next time you question your stress levels, don't wait until your body is telling you about it through physical tension – pay attention to the smaller physical adjustments and unhelpful changes in the way you think and feel on an emotional level, too.

Note: exercise should not get in the way of social events. It is a tool that keeps you mentally and physically healthy. Some people have a tendency to become dependent on it to excessive degrees. This results in a disturbance in mood and can worsen both physical and mental health. Overtraining is recorded as being the cause of deep depressions in some of the world's most famous athletes.

This mental health workout relies on your motives for exercising being healthy rather than part of an attempt to escape (such as in exercise addictions or eating disorders). Seeing as I am in recovery from an eating disorder, along with the body dysmorphia that comes with that, and to anyone reading this who is in the same position, it remains important that we do not exercise as an attempt to change our bodies. I work out in ways that I enjoy because it feels good, not because I want my body to be anything other than what it is.

When I consult with personal trainers I ask them to look out for two things as signals that someone's mind is suffering at the hands of exercise:

1. **Inconsistencies in energy levels** Any major energy highs or lows. Pay close attention to this – it might be your mind trying to protect your body or vice versa.

2. **Exercising on any type of injury** If you feel you cannot stop exercising, even though you are injured or poorly or tired, we have a problem.

If you recognise yourself in either of these scenarios, whether in the past or at any point in the future, please take it as a signal and give yourself permission to stop, rest and figure out a more healthy and helpful approach for you.

To conclude, cardiovascular exercise alone is beneficial to your mental health, but we have also explored ways of making your physical workout much more of a mental health workout. You can really make your three weekly sessions work for you by exploring both what your body needs and what your mind responds best to. Over time, exercise is the mental health workout that you can layer into your other workouts to experience huge emotional and psychological benefits.

YOUR MENTAL HEALTH WORKOUT WEEKLY CHECKLIST

WEEKLY WORKOUTS	M	T	W	TH	F	S	SU
THERAPY							
SOCIAL EVENTS							
EXERCISE							
SELF-CARE							

DAILY WORKOUTS							
MINDFULNESS							
CONNECTION							
APPRECIATION							
MOVEMENT							

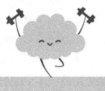

4 x Self-care

Last on your weekly programme is self-care – and this is the weekly workout that requires the most focus from you. It is essential because self-care, in return for your hard work, fills you up with vitality and progresses your psychological stamina – the ability to sustain a prolonged physical or mental effort. And embarking on a 5-week plan certainly requires that!

Building an effective self-care practice takes time and effort, and from a mental health perspective, it's about working both internally and externally to develop the specific muscles in question (similar to the visible and invisible work you did with your range of motion on pp. 54–5).

In this workout, we will break down both forms of self-care and guide you to make this a progressive exercise, as it is highly likely that over the next five weeks, as your stamina increases, you'll feel encouraged to come back to this workout and enrich it.

Many of us have blocks to authentically looking after ourselves. These emotional blocks build up over time and inhibit us from developing the stamina we want and need.

So I'd like to start by giving you an extra warm-up exercise to help clear these. If you ever have trouble with self-care, this is a great workout to come back to as a modification. There is also some extra help with clearing emotional blockages in the physio section (see p. 200).

Self-care warm-up exercise

Repeat the following to yourself three times in a row each day:

- 'When I embrace the concept of self-care, I release myself from the belief that I am, in any way, unlovable.'

You can change the words to suit you. Some variations include:

- 'When I accept self-care, I let go of the thought that I am unlovable.'
- 'I release myself from the belief that I am unlovable by letting self-care in.'

The intention behind this is to help you to become willing to shift any emotional blockages that might get in the way of you developing an effective self-care workout.

SELF-CARE WORKOUT

2 x external:

1. Identify things that make you feel good.

2. Decide which of these are healthy treats and distractions.

3. Make sure to plan them into your week.

2 x internal:

1. Work on your internal conversation with yourself.

2. Listen in, be honest, be brave, be kind and committed.

3. Make sure you plan this time into your week too.

WHY WE DO THIS WORKOUT

Self-care has become a bit of a mental health mainstay for many of us over the past few years, helping countless people to concentrate on themselves in what has become a very busy and unpredictable world. Social networking platforms have allowed the self-care movement to flourish and have given us the content to consider what external self-care looks and feels like. What is often not often explained fully, however, is the importance of internal self-care and how the two interact to support your mental health. External self-care is important and does work, momentarily, but when that moment passes, we often experience a sense of lack, which leads to us wanting to consume the 'stuff' or 'do' the thing more and more. We then run the risk of falling into addictive patterns and further highlighting inequalities and imbalances, rather than achieving true connective healing.

Because of the specialities I've trained in – addiction and trauma – I've worked with a plethora of clients who really struggle, fundamentally, to look after themselves. Hence, I've developed an excellent eye for the subtleties of self-care. Over the years, as I've worked with more and more people from all sorts of backgrounds – those who come to me when they are at rock bottom with their addictions and mental health issues and those who come because they want to realign with themselves or to identify the roadblock to fulfilling their potential – I have noticed that the universal struggle is not necessarily that we are not looking after ourselves, but that we lack the insight and effort required to create a self-care routine that looks after us, inside and out.

Part of the problem is that we are mainly exposed to inspiration for external self-care which can cost money, contributing to the messaging that money = happiness. In addition, much of the 'self-care industry' is appearance- and beauty-focused, aiming to make you feel better about your outsides, conveying yet another message – that attractive = happy. So we do this workout to target your insides, so that you can be happy with whatever reasonable state your outsides are in.

We also do this workout because, contrary to what the media would sometimes have us believe, the power we find in self-care does not come from the action itself but from the resulting feelings and behaviours. As an example, I love long baths as a form of external self-care; afterwards I feel relaxed, quiet and calm – an indication that my nervous system is happy and unstressed. From this happy and unstressed place, I am much more likely to feel empowered and motivated in my life in general. The bath is simply a tool in the self-care process rather than self-care itself.

Having said that, your self-care workout is not about changing how you feel, although it will do that; it is about supporting and motivating yourself via compassion as demonstrated in the example above, rather than pushing and punishing yourself to make yourself change, which is unsustainable. We do this workout because it fuels your mind and gives you the strength and stamina for the rest of your programme – and the rest of your life. We also do it because it influences the intensity you can tolerate and your endurance throughout. Done well, self-care stops you coasting and encourages organic progression within Your Mental Health Workout.

A CLOSER LOOK AT SELF-CARE

Being a radical self-care advocate, I believe it is important and helpful for us to understand what the self-care movements we choose are contributing to. It's a technique thing, if nothing else – when you understand how the muscle works, you know better how to move it in order to create the result you are looking for.

In the daily workouts, we will explore in more detail the ins and outs of your internal world, but for now, I want to familiarise you with the details of both external and internal self-care.

External self-care

External self-care movements are a bit like visible boundaries. In fact, the boundaries warm-up (see p. 48) was preparing you for this main self-care workout. External self-care is the type that is visible from the outside. It is first about self-soothing and it works in those emotionally distressing moments when we are stressed, anxious and scared, when our minds go offline and we can't think, or when our feelings are so strong that we feel like they have the capacity to take us under. Those of you who have ever experienced anxiety or panic attacks will immediately understand the importance of this.

External self-care also allows you to soothe yourself when you are in any physical pain or when you are poorly. Your external self-care movements should feel comforting and empowering and allow your nervous system to regain balance. They are also a distraction: you change your focus by diverting yourself from your inside world through something in your outside world. We often demonise 'distractions', but they can be very helpful. They are part of a rather clever and protective denial system that allows us to regulate our intake of information at a pace that we can cope with. We all have suffering, we all have pain and we all need distractions to help us tolerate our individual difficulties; if we did not have distractions or denial, lots more of us would find the reality of life incredibly difficult to function in.

There is another type of external self-care that comes from a place of self-worth, love and esteem and we do not need to be in emotional distress to practise it. When we do nice things for ourselves, we fuel and power up the message that we care, and we are more likely to do it again as we feel empowered by it. This also, in tandem, supports core stability, empowering us to make good choices for ourselves going forward. Take a moment here to remind yourself of the self-esteem warm-up we did (see p. 45) – this is one of the things it was preparing you for.

It's up to you which activities you choose to define your external self-care. Part of the workout is experimenting and finding what works for you, rather than doing things that may or may not have been effective for someone else. Your personalised external self-care is the fuel that gives you the space to consider *and then do* the internal work.

Just to get you thinking, here are a few of my favourite external self-care activities:

- Long, hot baths
- Hot drinks in a big mug
- Getting an early night
- Going for walks
- Music
- Reading fiction
- Having a lazy day
- Exercise
- Meditation
- Sticking to a sleep hygiene routine
- Journaling
- Phoning a friend, with or without a reason

MENTAL HEALTH MYTH

'Self-care is selfish'

You probably thought I was going to say 'self-care is not selfish', but, a bit controversially, I am going to tell you that self-care *is* selfish. However, it is selfish in a good way. We tend to define selfishness as being devoted to or caring only for oneself; concerned primarily with one's own interests, benefits, welfare, etc., regardless of others. But my argument is that it is not always a negative state to be experiencing. True, we don't want it to become a permanent trait or a way of life, but the prescriptive nature of Your Mental Health Workout allows you to carve out time in your week to be a bit selfish and experiment with how you can best fuel yourself through self-care.

So go ahead and be selfish with your self-care workout. Don't worry yourself with what others think about it; and if someone alludes to the fact that what you are doing is selfish, simply agree with them and let them know when you will be available for future unselfish interactions.

Internal self-care

Internal self-care is about starting the conversation with the vulnerable parts of you – the parts that you don't let anyone else see. Do you remember in your therapeutic-space workout we talked about the parts of your emotional and psychological world as being equivalent to different body parts you might work on at the gym? Well, we are using a similar concept here, except now you are working on those parts in your own time, outside of your therapeutic space too.

Internal self-care is about having those difficult conversations with yourself: the sad moments, the lonely nights and vulnerable experiences that make up part of your mental health muscle (feelings). It is also your internal cheerleader and complements both the core-stability warm-up and the appreciation workout in the daily section (see pp. 36 and 170, respectively). This is how you build strength from the inside, rather than the definition that you can show off to others.

Believe it or not, it is the practice of having these uncomfortable conversations with ourselves and learning to cheer ourselves on that allows us to have uncomfortable conversations with others and support them authentically. So the more practised we are at internal self-care, the more likely we are to be able to bust the stigma and judgment outside of ourselves. Although it is private, internal self-care done well contributes to wider change.

A bit like those invisible boundaries we worked on in the warm-up, this is a type of self-care that others do not and cannot see, and it can't be shared in the same way as external self-care. It can feel frustrating to not get that external validation through posting on social media, looking great or spending money, but we are much more likely to feel whole, happy and healthy when we are able to tend to all the parts of ourselves through internal self-care on a regular basis.

When we've got our internal self-care in check, along with the external stuff, we are able to make really empowered and life-changing choices, consistently. The choices I refer to here are across the board – self-care has the power to change who you choose to be in a relationship with, what job you want to do, how you apply yourself and how you use your self-esteem and boundaries. It powers up your core stability and protects your range of motion to ultimately nourish your mental health. And the bonus is that this is the type of energy that people really enjoy being around. When you are well fuelled through internal self-care, we attract a similar type of energy and motivation which, in turn, creates countless windows of opportunity to further nourish your mind.

We are going to make your self-care practice something that is undoubtedly yours, something that empowers you and that you can count on. As we know, every body and every mind is slightly different, so what works for you will depend on your personal experiences, culture, privilege and unique nature.

A solid internal self-care practice can nourish you from the inside far more than a weekend at a spa or a new pair of shoes will do. It is like having all the gym kit you need right there with you all the time. Internal self-care balances out the inequalities and imbalances between humans because it understands that we are all fundamentally equal and that looking after ourselves is a right. When you come from a place of privilege, it can sometimes feel easier to stick with external self-care, as you have the resources to do so, but please know that by doing that you opt to have far less responsibility for the internal and more unconscious feelings, thoughts and behaviours that can often contribute to inequality in society. Also, exclusively using privilege or wealth to 'fix' things – be it situations, other people or, indeed, your own mental health – gives you the message that nothing works in the long run, and there must be something wrong with you, as you constantly need these short-term fixes; you never create and internalise the kit that works for you.

HOW TO GET THIS WORKOUT WORKING FOR YOU
Ask yourself the following questions.

1. How do you define self-care?

2. Why do you practise self-care?

3. What does self-care achieve for you when you do it?

4. What do you want to get out of your self-care practice?

It is important to distinguish between the last two questions in order to get this workout working for you and create your individualised self-care kit. Be honest with yourself: what does your current self-care 'workout' achieve for you? And what do you want to get out of it that you are not already?

You are going to have to put the hard work into creating

a self-care kit that is really effective for you; to get you started here are a few of my favourites:

- Positive internal self-talk.
- Resting (mental, emotional, physical and sensory).
- Sticking to the commitments I make to myself.
- Acknowledging what I feel to myself before sharing it with others.
- Allowing myself to not be on 'best form'.
- Not pressuring myself to use social media if I don't want to.
- Parenting my inner child.

To help you create your own internal self-care kit, I have broken down the steps I use into motivation, execution and hopefulness on the next page.

DISCOVERING SELF-CARE WORKOUT: CREATING YOUR SELF-CARE ACTIVITIES

Pick a self-care action you have engaged with recently or intend to engage with in the near future. It can be internal or external (it's usually easier to start with external).

1. **What is your *motivation* for doing the chosen self-care action?**

   - Is it about you?
   - Is it about someone else?
   - Is it about looking good?
   - Is it about feeling better?
   - Maybe it's about tuning into yourself?

2. **How do you plan to *execute* this self-care activity?**

   - What is your aim or plan?
   - How will you make this happen for you?

3. **How *hopeful* does this make you feel?**

   - Does the sum of your motivation and execution give you a sense of hopefulness?

- Does it leave you feeling empowered or powerless?
- Helpful or helpless?

If the sum of your motivation and execution creates a feeling of hope, then your chosen self-care activity is one that is likely to work for you and can be added to you kit.

If you do not feel hopeful, you might prefer to pick a different self-care activity, rather than force yourself to do something that does not ignite hope. You only want things in your kit that bring you hope and comfort.

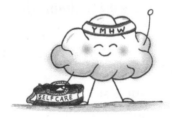

I hope this chapter and the workouts included in it have supported you in deepening your understanding of self-care. It matters much less what your self-care kit actually looks like and whether other people think it is selfish than what it helps you to connect with and feel. Feelings are the fuel; they are how we heal and what we must focus on.

As we come to the end of your weekly workout section, remind yourself once again of the goals you have set. Are you moving in that direction? Does anything need tweaking? Do you feel set up for success?

I would also suggest that now is a great time to take a

break, give yourself a breather and allow your mind to digest the information you've taken in . . . It's a lot! Take a day or two off, and spend some time journaling about what you have learned so far, including any hopes and fears that have come up, and plan your weekly workouts before moving on to the daily workouts in Chapter 5.

YOUR MENTAL HEALTH WORKOUT WEEKLY CHECKLIST

WEEKLY WORKOUTS	M	T	W	TH	F	S	SU
THERAPY							
SOCIAL EVENTS							
EXERCISE							
SELF-CARE							

DAILY WORKOUTS							
MINDFULNESS							
CONNECTION							
APPRECIATION							
MOVEMENT							

Chapter 5

YOUR DAILY MENTAL HEALTH WORKOUTS

— — — —

NOW THAT YOU'VE completed your weekly workouts and got most of your major mental health muscle groups moving, it's time to get a bit more internal and really sweaty with the daily work.

In this section of the programme, you will find your daily mental health workouts. They are designed to help you navigate your internal world with curiosity and ease. These are the ones that heal the injuries that no one else notices – those within your relationship with yourself. They build you up from the inside.

Remember, as always, planners and checklists are downloadable from www.yourmentalhealthworkout.com and you are welcome to use your separate journal to continue with the questions posed throughout.

Daily Workouts Explained

Your daily mental health workout programme looks like this:

1 x **Mindfulness** – hydrating your workout
2 x **Connection** – aerobic workout
3 x **Appreciation** – the finisher
4 x **Movement** – your cooldown

These are much smaller movements than the weekly workouts, and while many won't be noticeable to the outside eye, they create definition and contentment on the inside.

They target your self-concept (how you construct who you are and the beliefs you hold about yourself), self-talk and base levels of happiness. With a bit of practice, you can take these daily workouts anywhere with you and progress the weekly ones to include them when the time is right. It is this work that maintains the resilience, commitment, hope and love within yourself.

Over time, these, like the weekly workouts, become a way of life, rather than a daily checklist.

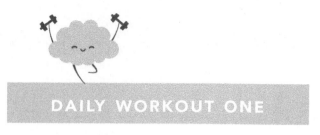

1 x Mindfulness

Mindfulness is the act of intentionally attending to the present moment without judgment or attachment. It is accepting this moment exactly as it is, and ourselves exactly as we are.

Your daily mindfulness workout is about staying present, aware, happy and healthy, and training your mind to focus on the things that help it, rather than hinder it.

FIRST, FIND YOUR MINDFUL HOLD

1. Pause what you are doing.

2. Observe what your body is doing right now. Focus on your breath. Where do you feel it most? Your nose? Your belly? Your chest?

3. You have just identified your mindful hold.

Your mindful hold is a resting position that gives you some-thing specific and feel-able to come back to each time you need a moment of mindfulness. It is an internal exercise that you can do anywhere.

MINDFULNESS WORKOUT

1. Assign a time each day. Maybe when you wake up, before you brush your teeth or after lunch, for example.

2. Set a time limit. Start with 1 or 2 minutes and, over the course of Your Mental Health Workout, increase the time as you progress.

3. Notice your breath – your mindful hold (see previous page). Don't change it; just notice what it is doing.

4. Notice your mental health muscle and its equipment just as they are right now.

5. Choose where you want your focus to be in this moment.

If you notice any feelings or thoughts that are pulling your focus, use one or both of the witnessing phrases below and then repeat steps 3–5:

'I am noticing I am having a thought that _____'

'I am noticing I am feeling _____ about _____'

WHY WE DO THIS WORKOUT

When I was first developing my ideas around the daily workouts I went backwards and forwards between mindfulness and meditation. Research dating back thousands of years proves to us that meditation is effective at calming and clearing the mind. But many of us, with our current busy lifestyles, find a classical meditation practice difficult to implement and stick to and I wanted to give you something that is realistically attainable and makes sense within your current lifestyle.

Meditation can be much more than sitting down with your eyes closed trying to clear your mind – movement, journaling, music, chanting can all be used as forms of meditation, and these days it has many crossovers with what we call mindfulness. In fact, most practitioners consider meditation to be just one part of a mindfulness journey. It is usually understood as a relaxation exercise, whereas mindfulness as a lifestyle is something slightly different.

We do this workout to help you pinpoint thought spirals that lead to unhappy emotional states; we do it to help you notice the judgments you cast upon yourself and others; and we do it to empower you to choose where your attention goes and where you hold your focus.

Consider mindfulness as the equivalent to hydrating your workout – pretty vital, wouldn't you say? It is a useful source of refreshment that is helpful to always have available. It is designed to help you feel calmer and more connected – better hydrated, within the context of our metaphor. So, we do this workout to keep you healthy during all this hard work and able to continue to grow through working with your feelings via developing a mindful authority over your thoughts, feelings and behaviours. Just as we can forget to drink enough water during a busy or mindless day, we are sometimes at emotional risk of getting busy or mindless and forgetting or avoiding opportunities to stop and take a sip of mindfulness. A lack of mindfulness can mean you don't realise how thirsty you are, emotionally, psychologically or, indeed, physically, so that you can end up seeming a bit absent-minded, forgetting things and making mistakes. For those who struggle to create space for themselves during busy days and demanding jobs: no one would stop you grabbing a glass of water, would they? So, give yourself the same permission to hydrate your mind by grabbing a mindful moment. It feels cooling and cleansing. You have to hydrate your body and mind in order to continue with the other parts of your workout.

Used alongside your weekly and other daily workouts, mindfulness has the capacity to transform your perspective, prevent mental health declines by helping you spot them sooner and create the space in your mind to make informed decisions on how you want to use your mental health muscle in general. We do it because it helps train our minds to avoid the autopilot mode that runs the show carelessly if we let it. It helps to keep us connected to ourselves by consistently being aware of our thoughts, feelings and behaviours and therefore giving us more emotional freedom in our day-to-day lives.

MENTAL HEALTH MYTH

'Mindfulness is about relaxing, being positive and having a clear mind'

Yes, mindfulness *can* be relaxing and refreshing, hence the hydration metaphor, and it might help clear your mind. But the outcome we are seeking here is for you to be able to choose where your focus goes – and when you have this type of authority over your focus you can then decide when and what takes precedence in your life and train your mind to think positively. But you absolutely do not have to; we are not trying to make pessimists into optimists or optimists into realists here – we are just trying to hold focus.

When exercising mindfulness it's important you are aware and noticing your thoughts and validating all types of thoughts and feelings, rather than trying to banish them (both thoughts and feelings can be a bit like boomerangs: the more force used to throw them away, the more force they come back with). Once you've noticed them, mindfully and without judgment, you can then choose what you'd like to do with them. You can take action . . . or not, if that's what you decide.

Why the mindful hold?

Your mindful hold – the thing we identified on p. 133 – helps create safety inside you. Your mindful hold is available to you always because it is part of you, and the more you use it, the easier it is to find. We point towards your breath because, well, lots of us hold our breath when we have difficult feelings and thoughts in an attempt to physically control our emotions, but breath is still there to guide you – it just gets pushed aside. The more you familiarise yourself with your breath and where it comes from – how you feel it, where you feel it (your mindful hold) – the more you can consciously direct your awareness to different parts of your workout (and life) and maintain that sense of feeling refreshed and hydrated throughout. You can use your mindful hold to relax tense reactions in your body and to give you some agency over the intensity of your feelings and, likewise, the stresses of everyday life.

Your mindful hold will assist you in identifying unhelpful use of your mental health equipment faster. Therapeutically, we call unhelpful changes in your thinking 'cognitive distortions' and, to keep the workout metaphor going strong, we are going to call them cognitive pulls, so you can think of them as something that pulls your mental health muscle (ouch!) away from where it needs to be.

Ten simple ways to practise mindfulness

1. Do a body scan (notice and name the sensations in each part of your body).

2. Notice where your breath is in your body.

3. Listen to the different noises around you.

4. Focus on something specific.

5. Focus on something soothing.

6. Slow down.

7. Validate your thoughts without judging.

8. Trust in this moment.

9. Adopt an attitude of self-acceptance.

10. Remain aware of your distractions.

HOW TO GET THIS WORKOUT WORKING FOR YOU

Mindfulness is easy to get lost with and can be difficult if we don't have an entry point. To get this working for you, I suggest you start to understand your cognitive pulls. It gives you something internal to be actively mindful about. You can, of course, apply the mindfulness workout to any external activity as well.

Understanding your cognitive pulls

Cognitive pulls develop as a way of getting you away from what's happening right now. They take you out of the present moment. Weirdly, sometimes, even though pulls tend to have an objectively negative bias, focusing as they do on negative thought patterns and core beliefs (and if they were muscular, they would be quite painful), they feel safer and 'better' than being in your reality, in your present moment. Mindfulness can help to neutralise your judgments and encourage you to navigate your thoughts with more compassion and ease to craft a much calmer path through your mental health journey.

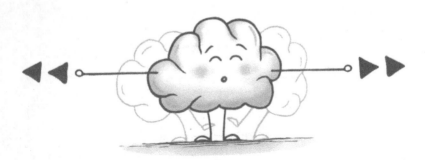

To help you get this workout working for you, I have identified nine pulls that have appeared in my consulting room over the years, explaining them in very basic forms. In the first instance, have a read through them and see what you identify with. Then, see which of them you notice when engaging with your mindfulness workout and start to become an observer. You might notice that you have a preferred pull that you default to every time the present moment becomes too difficult or painful – similar to a muscular pull or a repetitive stress injury. You may also recognise yourself in all of them and identify that you feel pulled in many directions. Either way, it's helpful to know what you are working with.

Here are nine common cognitive pulls:

- **Catastrophising** is a particularly common cognitive pull because it makes sense to us, when we are stressed, upset or panicking, to plan for the worst-possible-case scenario. It is our minds' way of getting ready for battle. But, when the worst-possible scenarios become negative fantasies and intrusive thoughts and we get attached to them, they cause feelings of stress and anxiety and are extraordinarily unhelpful. This pull is more common than most because it comes in the exact opposite form as well, known as minimising.

- **Minimising** is when you tell yourself and others that it's not that bad – in fact, there is nothing wrong. This is the 'I'm-fine' syndrome. Both catastrophising (sometimes known as maximising) and minimising are forms of denial.

- **Denial** is more of a cognitive block than a pull, so to speak. It's a very clever mechanism that our minds use to help us regulate the input of information to a pace that works for us. However, denial can also cause mental health aches, pains and strains if we are constantly blocking out information about the present moment. Mindfulness can support you in becoming more aware of the things you deny in life, including your thoughts, feelings and behaviours.

- **Blaming/shaming** I put these together as one cognitive pull because they are, in my mind, one and the same; shame is blame turned inwards. With this cognitive pull, you are either shaming yourself harshly for something that has happened, or you are blaming others to avoid the unhelpful feelings that have probably lived inside you for much longer than you are aware. When you engage in blame on any level you make others responsible for your feelings, and – as if I have not said it enough already – you are responsible for your own feelings and that is a very good thing! It is my opinion that no one can *make* you feel anything unless you let them and vice versa. Knowing this will help you identify if you are struggling with this distorted way of thinking. Your daily mindfulness practice, alongside all the internal self-care work we just did (see pp. 123–125) allows you to start the practice of taking responsibility.

- **Polarisation** Yep, you guessed it, this way of thinking is all or nothing, black or white. Ironically, it is a way of thinking and behaving that is sometimes affirmed in many self-help and wellbeing communities that intend to motivate people to give their all. Statements like 'Go hard or go home', 'If you are not going to do it properly, why do it at all?' or, 'You showed up to work, why waste your time?' encourage this particular pull in those who do not yet know how to spot and manage it.

The reason we adopt polarisation is because these statements feel like a threat, and when we perceive a threat we jump into action; this cognitive pull is a misguided attempt to arouse motivation. The danger here is that we might feel that unless we visit the 'all' end of polarisation, which is created through external factors that might not have our wellbeing at heart, rather than a customised 'all' within which we function well, we believe we are a failure. Some will go to great lengths and chase what they think success looks like, while others will become afraid of the implied failure and do nothing instead. Mindfulness encourages you to consider that wherever you fall on the spectrum, within whatever you happen to be doing, that is just the present experience, and it does not need to be altered in any way. Mindfulness helps you become OK with the middle ground.

- **Perfectionism** This is very much part of the polarisation distortion, but a specific form of it. There is nothing wrong with using other people, places and things to motivate yourself to be better, and it is totally OK for you to have high standards for yourself. Having said that, dangerous levels of perfectionism are on the rise when you are setting standards that you can't meet. Perfect does not exist.

143

Perfect is the goalpost that you think you are going
to reach, when you think you are going to feel
gratified by achieving a particular grade or hitting a
certain financial or social goal, but when you get
there (and a perfectionist will always get there) it
feels disappointing and not quite as validating as you
expected it to. So the perfectionism cognitive pull
moves the goalposts, and you'll feel like you never
made it in the first place, it's all an illusion.

- **Generalising** This is when you make a sweeping
  assumption about things based on a single experience.
  For example, you see someone wearing a hat and
  doing something silly and you take this to mean that
  all people who wear hats are silly. This pull is
  unhelpful because it tends (like the others) to have a
  negative bias, so that if something bad happens once,
  your mind expects it to happen over and over again.
  Generalising can contribute to a feeling of never-
  ending defeat if we are not mindful about it.

- **Personalisation** is a way of thinking that tells
  you everything is about you. This usually does not
  work in your favour as it has a direct negative
  consequence on your core stability. If you experience
  a personalisation pull, you will always be comparing
  yourself and trying to control what other people
  think and feel about you, and you might feel that
  you caused negative events which, in fact, had
  nothing to do with you. In this particular scenario,

mindfulness helps you to notice the things that are happening outside of yourself that contribute to how situations play out. It allows you to be less self-focused and more realistic about your part in events.

- **Filtering** This is a way of thinking that only focuses on one detail, and that detail is sometimes taken out of context too. If you experience this pull, you'll often ignore other important parts of your reality. The really common one you might identify with is when 99 out of 100 people think you are wonderful, while the other one seems disinterested or to think badly of you. You then focus on that one person's view and base your beliefs about yourself on that, rather than on those of the other 99 who absolutely respect you and have your back.

JOURNAL OPPORTUNITY: COGNITIVE PULLS IN ACTION

Do you see yourself in any of the cognitive pulls described above? Explain.

Are you aware of any other pulls that we haven't named already?

We usually find that these negative thought cycles and cognitive pulls are exaggerated when something difficult is going on and we don't want it to be happening to us. In other words, we are not happy with our present moment and are trying to find ways to change it. Our focus stays on the negative and creates a negativity bias that kicks in when we feel under threat. The consequence is that we then move further away from our reality, further away from the present moment and create additional levels of anxiety.

Knowing your personal cognitive pulls and their distinct intensities, and actively applying your mindfulness workout accordingly is how you get this working for you. Just notice. Don't judge, don't compare. This is about being curious in yourself.

Over time, as your mindful muscle matures through daily use, mindfulness will become easier and more effective, and you will have the sense of authority over your thoughts and feelings that I have been talking about throughout the programme so far. And its effectiveness never stops increasing because each time you do it, it will be different – you'll notice other thoughts and feelings, become aware of your less conscious processes and feel increasingly calmer and stronger.

YOUR MENTAL HEALTH WORKOUT WEEKLY CHECKLIST

WEEKLY WORKOUTS	M	T	W	TH	F	S	SU
THERAPY							
SOCIAL EVENTS							
EXERCISE							
SELF-CARE							

DAILY WORKOUTS							
MINDFULNESS							
CONNECTION							
APPRECIATION							
MOVEMENT							

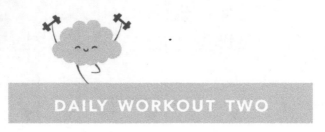

2 x Connection

You have taken in a lot of information so far and I hope trying out the mindfulness workout has allowed you to stay focused and digest those big workouts in the weekly section. At this point, please remember it is always OK to take breaks when you need them. In fact, I support you 100 per cent in taking a mindful breather as and when you need to.

Your connection workout is the equivalent to the aerobic section of your physical programme. It can get your heart rate up a little and make you 'sweat'. It gets you a bit out of breath and includes the majority of the difficult movements we've worked on so far.

CONNECTION WORKOUT

I want you to focus on connection in two ways, with yourself and then with others.

1 x self-connection workout

1. Each morning, before you do anything else, check in with your mental health muscle. Ask yourself: how am I feeling? (Use the 'foundation feelings' chart on pp. 14–5 to help you with this.)

2. Once you have identified how you are feeling, ask yourself: how am I going to work with that today?

3. Assess first what you need and then what you want from today.

4. Make a commitment to stay connected to yourself and work with, rather than against, your needs and wants for the next twenty-four hours. Make a new commitment each day.

1 x connection with others workout

1. Assess what you need and want from others on a daily basis.

2. Get to know your triggers.

3. Be conscious of your attachment styles.

4. Actively connect with others daily by making contact and listening – to understand rather than to respond. Ask them questions and feel free to state your point of view without trying to change the other person – connection is reciprocal.

Connection is a very active process, and it takes energy and commitment to do it daily. If you would like to progress this workout, simply double up: self-connect morning and evening and connect with others twice each day.

WHY WE DO THIS WORKOUT

We do this workout because ruptures in how we connect with ourselves and others are what have the most damaging effect on our core stability and range of motion. In fact, they have so much of an effect on our mental health that in psychology we often refer to these injuries as traumas. When there is a connection trauma, or disturbance, whether a death, a break-up, a disruptive move, bullying, abuse, a divorce or anything else you'd like to add, we don't stop trying to connect to others. In fact, we often develop a desperate yearning for relationships with others in an attempt to replace the connection that has been ruptured – and we lose our connection to ourselves. The conscious and unconscious insecurities and self-loathing that follow can lead to a desire to shut others out – and when that happens, not only do we feel discon-nected from ourselves, we also feel disconnected from others. Most of us find ways of seeking healing in this department because we are biologically built for connection. Sadly, when we seek repair in other people before reconnecting with ourselves it is like exercising on an injury and we often get hurt again. The only way to cope with this is to disconnect from ourselves, our feelings, our pain and our reality . . . again. We do this workout to heal our connection traumas with ourselves as well as others.

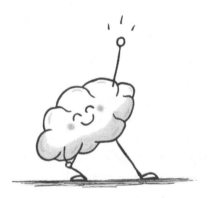

*'Trauma has to be an identifiable and catastrophic event
to cause the post-traumatic negative effects'*

We all experience trauma. Trauma, in my book, is anything less than helpful or any adverse experience that has happened in your life. This could be a major event, but it could also be hundreds of small disappointments, moments of feeling neglected and rejected. Your trauma is anything that has been unhelpful to you as an individual, and no two people will respond to trauma in the same way, even if they experience the same one.

You may or may not develop symptoms of post-traumatic stress disorder (PTSD). These days, we understand that PTSD shows up in any moment where your mind repeats (or believes it is repeating) a traumatic event. Most people, if you dig deep enough, have something like this with within their relational history that has hurt them enough to result in a PTSD response. A good example is when someone repeatedly gets into neglectful or abusive relationships and finds themselves wondering why they can't find love. It is their PTSD from historic connection injuries running the show, believing that it can heal itself by putting the person in the same situation over and over, each time believing that 'this time will be different'. But, in fact, it is just worsening an injury that is already too painful to cope with. Once you know this, and spot it in your life, you can start to gather the strength, through connecting and caring for yourself, to walk away from events that trigger PTSD responses.

Please also note that this can show up in any type of relationship, be it romantic, parental, with work colleagues, friends, siblings, authority figures, etc.

The damage done when connection ruptures shows up in many forms. Addictions, along with eating, identity and attachment disorders all thrive when we fall out of connection, regardless of the reason. They thrive because we are trying to heal ourselves, by finding something to connect with, and we mistake these behaviours for something that makes us feel safe and loved. They are misconnections with ourselves, however, and the longer we exercise on them the more painful they get in the long run.

So, we do this workout to start healing our misconnections with ourselves and also to practise what it feels like to allow ourselves to depend on and connect with others. Research demonstrates that in any situation where humans come together, feeling connected with and developing a strong community with like-minded people supports wellbeing. When we feel included and supported by a community, we meet our basic human need for belonging. We experience less loneliness and are less likely to withdraw and isolate ourselves. We become physically healthier, with stronger immune systems and lower stress levels.

Feeling seen, witnessed and heard for who we are and all our wants and needs heals our minds, as well as our bodies. We do this workout so that we know exactly what it is we want and need to be seen, witnessed and heard. We do it to protect ourselves from loneliness because if we become too lonely, the need deepens and, eventually, reaching out to others becomes too risky, the risk of further rejection becomes intolerable and we shut down on ourselves. Again.

This is a very easy workout to back away from because it highlights the parts of ourselves that are hurt and have been rejected or left unloved, and our natural instinct is to move away from pain, not towards it. It also challenges us to face painful feelings like loneliness and shame and to become vulnerable for the sake of our health. It also starts to provide some muscle mass, as well as psychological strength, stamina and flexibility from the inside.

There can be some confusion about how much we should be connecting with and relying on ourselves versus depending on others. I can make this very simple for you: in an emergency, you need to be able to self-regulate via connection to yourself. Those who do not work on this might experience higher levels of anxiety, depression and be prone to the aforementioned addictive behaviours. So we need to strengthen that part of you enough and ensure that you are connected with and feel you can support yourself. However, it is actually proven that the nervous system regulates itself better when it is with someone else – hence the importance of being able to authentically connect with others too and get your needs and wants met.

There is sometimes further confusion about the difference between connection, communication and attachment, all of which are key parts of this workout. Eventually, you might like to progress your connection workout with yourself and other people to focus specifically on one or all of these three things.

- **Connection** = a reciprocal and emotionally driven relationship in which one or more needs and wants are being met. Feels like: you are able to hold your core stability and use your range of motion well.

- **Communication** = the act of conveying what you need and want. Feels like: a strengthening of your core stability and a test of your range of motion.

- **Attachment** = often stems from unmet childhood needs that have become insatiable in adulthood. Feels like: desperation and a yearning that will never be met.

We do this workout to help you navigate the very potent and painful feelings that come up in relationships, whether it's a connection, communication or attachment concern.

HOW TO GET THIS WORKOUT WORKING FOR YOU
This workout asks that you put effort into understanding yourself and managing your internal responses to others. To do that, you need:

- a handle on your psychological triggers
- to connect with yourself via your wants and needs
- an understanding of your attachment style
- connection with others.

Know your trigger points

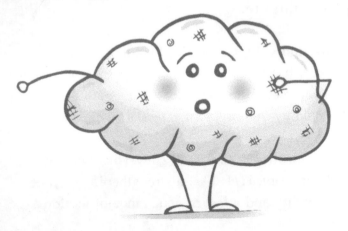

On your body you have a number of 'trigger points'. Different for everyone, these are areas that feel tender and respond to pressure without you having to tell them what to do. They often cause pain. Your mind also has a set of triggers that have been created over time, through your experiences in relationships. Understanding your individual triggers – where they come from and why they bother you – is the best way to get this workout working for you.

When triggered, we often find ourselves disconnecting from our reality and abandoning and disconnecting from ourselves to cope. This can look like completely freezing and shutting down or seeing red and going into a rage, as well as anything in between. In the moment, you lose your choice about how you react, your feelings ignite and all your cognitive pulls activate.

Triggers can be internal, in the shape of thoughts and feelings, or external, in the shape of people, places and things – like a smell or a song that reminds you of something. The memories activated internally or externally are often referred to as flashbacks. Trigger points are specific to your experience, and the original catalyst does not have to be present for your feelings and thoughts to dominate and overwhelm you.

Familiarising yourself with your psychological trigger points

1. Make a list of things that happen this week that trigger you. Use the definition above to help you.

2. Create safety for yourself by removing your contact with any external triggers for now and, if you are able to identify the internal ones, start noticing when they are likely to occur by logging them in your planner or journal.

3. When triggered by people, places and things, or indeed thoughts and feelings use your mindful hold to self-soothe and hydrate your system back to balance (see p. 133).

There will be days where you feel super-capable, strong, flexible and able to care for yourself when your trigger points are activated. And there will be days when you'll need to be much gentler because, for whatever reason – tiredness, hormones, other life events – you are already close enough to your psychological edge. As you develop the skills of connection, you will be able to call in support in the form of your therapeutic space and social events or, in the absence of those, use your mindfulness workout (cooling and cleansing – see p. 134) to help you tune into what you need on any given day.

Over time, and when you are in good connection to yourself and others, you may be able to interact with things that used to trigger you without experiencing the rush of emotion. If you do get to a point where you'd like to reintroduce the person, place or thing that triggers you, do it slowly and pay even closer attention to your self-connection workout.

Learn to connect with yourself via your wants and needs
The second part of getting this workout working for you is the self-connection part. Self-connection is all about tuning in with thoughts, feelings and behaviours and using them to guide you to recognise need and want and distinguish between the two.

Those of you who have ever suffered with addictions, eating disorders or self-destructive acts have an advantage here. The cravings that can occur with these compulsive behaviours are an excellent barometer for when you are about to or have already fallen out of connection with yourself – as long as you do not act out on the compulsion, of course. For those have not acted out in the same way, please note that sometimes we disconnect from ourselves in more subtle ways – like putting other people first a bit too much, not paying attention to our own wants or needs, not being able to say 'no' and not asking for help.

Connecting with yourself is a lifelong practice. You can start at any age, and it will serve you well in years to come. It can feel a bit fragile and getting this part of the workout working for you can take some trial and error – usually in the form of giving yourself something you thought you wanted, then realising when you get it that you needed something different. A classic example is when you eat on your feelings: you think you want to munch on sweet stuff, and meet that want by allowing yourself such snacks, only to feel disappointed when you've finished – because what you actually needed was to reach out, connect and get some emotional nurturing from someone who loves you.

- **Wants** = the things that bring you joy in life and improve your day-to-day happiness.
- **Needs** = the things you need to function physically or emotionally.

 JOURNAL OPPORTUNITY:
ASSESS YOUR NEEDS AND WANTS

How many basic needs are you meeting in your life right now?

- Are you eating healthily and in a balanced way?
- Are you drinking enough water?
- Do you have adequate living conditions and clothes to wear?
- How is your sleep hygiene?
- Do you feel safe?
- Do you have security in your relationships and job?
- Do you have strong friendships?
- Do you feel you belong?

- Are you working towards your goals and putting effort into your life?

What are your wants and how many of them are you meeting?
- What things bring you joy?
- What helps you feel connected to yourself?
- What are the things you do to reward yourself?
- Do you currently feel deprived?

Here's a tip: you will only feel awkward about meeting your wants if you are not already meeting all of your needs. Start connecting with yourself by meeting your needs and progress on to your wants.

Eight ways to connect with yourself

1. Check in with your feelings each morning.

2. Journal your thoughts.

3. Know the difference between wants and needs.

4. Identify your wants and needs.

5. Create time each day that is just for you.

6. Take your time.

7. Look into your own eyes daily, what do you see?

8. Touch your own body in a loving way (hugs, strokes, self-massage, etc.).

Understanding your attachment style

We've talked about the difference between connection, communication and attachment. Understanding your attachment style is another chance to get this workout working for you. Consider the descriptions below and underline the statements you identify with. For the purpose of this exercise, the words 'others' and 'relationship' can apply to any kind of attempted connection – friends, family, lovers, colleagues, partners, etc. You might also spot yourself in more than one or notice that you fall into different attachment styles within different types of relationship. The point of knowing about your attachment styles is that you can then exercise effective, internal self-care in relationship to the feelings that arise. For example, you might identify with avoidant attachments in romantic relationships, in which case you'll need to be gentle working with your fear of intimacy and developing a sense of spontaneity. And at the same time, you may relate to having a disorganised attachment style in relationships to, say, parents or authority figures – in which case the feelings to be focusing on would be anger and fear. Becoming conscious of the potential differences tells you what you need to be working on and helps you to connect with yourself so that you can then connect with others in a secure and happy way.

Secure attachment:
- You feel happy when you are around others.
- You feel protected and supported in general.
- You feel upset when separated from your significant others.
- Although you feel upset you are sure you will see your significant other again.
- You trust that your needs will be met.

Anxious attachment:
- You experience separation anxiety.
- You are not comforted in the presence of others.
- You do not feel able to rely on others.
- You often feel anxious, insecure and low-level angry or resentful in your relationships.
- You need consistent reassurance from others.

Avoidant attachment:
- You tend to keep away from others.

- You have a fear of intimacy.
- You tend to be emotionally distant.
- You struggle with spontaneity.
- You do not believe your needs will be met.
- You may have experienced abuse or neglect.

Disorganised attachment:
- You often feel confused and angry.
- You may have experienced a frightened or frightening caregiver connection.
- You have no strategy for meeting your own needs.
- You might experience dissociative episodes (where you detach from reality and lose time without realising).
- You might experience depression.

New research shows that we can indeed change our attachment styles as adults with a bit of willingness and hard work. I have included some suggested further reading on attachment on p. 227–230.

Connecting with others

In my experience, it is this moment in this workout that brings on the most fear for people – as if we've turned the speed knob up to high on the treadmill: they get scared, freak out and just stop. Their fear is not actually of connection, however – it is of separation; they are not scared of the pace, intimacy or commitment, but of the abandonment, pain or injury they make themselves vulnerable to. Get this workout working for you by looking through the statements below and challenging them by reaching out and connecting with others anyway.

I do not want to/cannot connect with others because:
- I don't want to be a burden.
- I can't be bothered.
- I am too boring/not interesting enough.
- People don't care.
- I don't need to; I am self-sufficient.
- What if they don't want to connect with me?
- I am awkward on the phone.
- No one answers their phone these days.
- I don't like people.
- People don't like me.
- They have nothing to give me.
- I have nothing to give them.
- I feel embarrassed.
- I feel like a disappointment.
- I feel unwanted.
- I don't need other people.

Each statement that you identified with, or if you added any of your own, believe it or not, gives you an indication as to exactly how to get connecting with others working for you. For example, if you identified with 'I can't be bothered', 'I am too boring' or 'People don't care', it is likely that you did not have attachment figures that showed enough interest in you and you have now internalised this as a lack of interest in yourself and assume others will not be bothered with you either. So, your work here involves changing your internal attachment narrative to the exact opposite. For example, 'I am an interesting person', 'I have people who care about me', 'I CARE ABOUT ME!' We will develop these further in the Appreciation workout (see p. 170). And yes, you might have to 'fake it until you make it' with the internal work here.

Eight ways to connect with others

1. Smile more and practise eye contact.

2. Express your wants and needs.

3. Let go of expectations.

4. Stick to your commitments – these include your boundaries.

5. Respect their boundaries.

6. Work on your empathy.

7. Be curious about the other person.

8. See all people as valuable, vulnerable and imperfect.

MENTAL HEALTH MYTH

'We attract what we deserve'

It is just not that simple. Trauma attracts trauma. It is something that has happened to you that was outside of your control and it changed you in ways you did not ask for. You did nothing to deserve the mental health scars that you carry, regardless of how you got them.

We attract and repeat what we know in an attempt to heal our psychological wounds. When you realise that you deserve more than repeating your history, you get to create the change you want. We attract what we are ready for.

Without connection our mental health declines rapidly. So, get this workout working for you by actively seeking connection with yourself, familiarising yourself with your trigger points, understanding your attachment style and pursuing connection with others, even when the fear of rejection or loneliness tries to hold you back.

The results of this workout move you towards a feeling of being loved and loving. When you do it on a daily basis you get the message that you are valuable, worthy, lovable and wanted. This, in turn, helps you to feel aligned, balanced, equal and worthy; yes, it actively supports your core stability and allows you to continue to like – or even love – yourself when you make mistakes and when you don't feel so great.

It is the feeling of connection, firstly with yourself and then with others, that allows you to cope with current or historic toxic experiences of abandonment, rejection, shame and loneliness – because when we feel connected, we know where to go to get our needs and wants met, whether from within ourselves or from others, and therefore we are able to orientate ourselves in a rather confusing world; we are no longer lost.

YOUR MENTAL HEALTH WORKOUT WEEKLY CHECKLIST

WEEKLY WORKOUTS	M	T	W	TH	F	S	SU
THERAPY							
SOCIAL EVENTS							
EXERCISE							
SELF-CARE							

DAILY WORKOUTS							
MINDFULNESS							
CONNECTION							
APPRECIATION							
MOVEMENT							

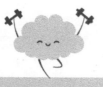

DAILY WORKOUT THREE

3 x Appreciation

At this point in your programme, you will be feeling the 'mental sweat' that has been building up. You've worked on your core, your range of motion, your endurance and overall mental fitness. Now, just like a physical workout, Your Mental Health Workout needs a finisher to get you that post-workout glow that looks good on everyone – even if *you* think you are sweaty mess.

This appreciation workout is your finisher.

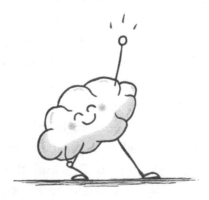

APPRECIATION WORKOUT

1. Pick three things, daily, that you are grateful for in your external or internal world.

2. Write them down. Vary them as much as possible.

3. Choose an affirmation for each day. For example, 'I am healing' or 'I deserve love' (see p. 176 for further examples). Repeat it to yourself in the mirror three times (you can increase the repetitions as you progress).

WHY WE DO THIS WORKOUT

We do this workout to help us move through the limitations we put on our own happiness and we do it to create love for ourselves. On a personal note, over the years, I have found this to be fundamental to my daily mental health hygiene. It has created an openness for change within me, helpful self-talk and a sturdy self-concept. It also helps me to understand that my potential in life is only constrained by the limitations I choose to put on it. That doesn't mean I am going to be able to fly one day, but it does mean that I feel empowered to manifest exactly what I need and want out of life and therefore to stay connected to myself. It is appreciation – 3 x gratitudes and 3 x affirmations per day – that I can credit with keeping me in good psychological shape. We do this workout so you can experience the same.

Gratitudes and affirmations are your finisher. A finisher always comes at the end of your workout and involves bursts of intensity to build more strength and endurance in the long term. It is important that you understand that although you could use this workout as a stand-alone exercise (and many people do), the reason many of us find gratitudes and affirmations difficult or ineffective is because, just like a physical workout finisher, they need to be done alongside the other workouts covered so far.

It can *look* like developing a positive mindset is the easiest things in the word – but it's not that simple and can be very frustrating for those of us who are unfamiliar, untrained or out of practice.

Affirmations and gratitudes are a challenge smothered with compassion, and they are much more than just creating a positive outlook on life. We do this workout because it has a profound effect on your self-concept by adjusting the script you hold about yourself.

Historically, how we develop and create our self-concept has been based on things like gender, sexuality and race; however, over the past few decades, we have moved into an arena that allows us to define ourselves exactly how we choose. This has resulted in the image and definition we have for ourselves being at once more fragile, yet more malleable. We get to decide who we want to be, and this workout helps to protect those decisions, and change them where necessary.

Because the appreciation workout affects something so

fundamental – your self-concept – and how you understand yourself and live your life, we sometimes experience a negative emotional response when we first start practising it.

Depending on your history, your response can happen at various levels of intensity in the form of self-criticism and feelings of shame, sadness and anger. As an example, you might write three perfectly lovely gratitudes and then get a voice in the back of your mind telling you that you don't deserve to be grateful, or that those gratitudes are not good enough. Another example: you might use an affirmation for the first time and then get a backlash from your internal chatter in the form of self-loathing and unhelpful intrusive thoughts. These responses, regardless of their intensity are simply down to the fact that no one has fully explained why we do these psychological movements and what you can expect from them, so naturally, having seen the positivity others put on them, you expect to feel positive, too. It is also worth mentioning that you might indeed have a very positive and immediate reaction, which is a good thing, and deepening your understanding of 'why' that happens will be what you gain out of doing this workout.

With all that in mind, we do this workout, daily, as part of Your Mental Health Workout to help you adjust, hone and protect your self-concept and practise the mental gymnastics that appreciation can be. This is where you gain your post-workout glow.

HOW TO GET GRATITUDE WORKING FOR YOU

Gratitude is the first part of your appreciation workout. It is proven that gratitude changes the way people make decisions and enables change. It is a big contributor to the post-workout glow – an indication of the empowerment, vitality and newly tapped energy that fire up your potential and your happiness. Gratitude is also probably the most talked about exercise in terms of mental health. In fact, I cannot think of a programme or model that does not endorse it as a way to support health and happiness.

It is true that some people are naturally more grateful than others. If you suffer from mental health problems, or have a tendency to self-destruct, you probably find your focus naturally falls on to the things in life that feel hard and those you do not have. The gratitude part of this workout attempts to flip that on its head: it makes you very aware of what privileges you *do* have in your life, creating a conscious focus on what is going right and leaving you with a post-workout glow on a daily basis, whatever your circumstances.

Through practising gratitude, you start acknowledging yourself and become willing to see the definition created in your self-concept through all the mental health workouts you've done so far. You can express gratitude for something internal like a talent or a trait or a passion. Or maybe you feel seen, you feel witnessed and you feel esteemed by yourself from the inside, when you acknowledge the things you have available to you in life – like your home, the food you eat and the people around you. When you express gratitude for things outside of yourself you are also acknowledging the things that bring you joy and invite them in.

Get gratitude working for you by ensuring you do it consistently enough. Keep in mind that change happens when the novelty wears off and you have to put the effort in.

Get gratitude working for you by including a minimum of three gratitudes per day. You are welcome to add or modify as you see fit – maybe you'd like to do three internal gratitudes (for yourself) and three external (for others) each day. Or maybe you'll increase the repetitions and do the workout twice a day, by either repeating or extending your list.

How you develop your gratitude practice is entirely up to you. I have found the old-fashioned way – a handwritten list – or sharing my gratitude with someone I love each day works best for me.

Some technical pointers on getting gratitude working for you

1. Become observant: notice what is going on right now; notice what privileges you have.

2. Let it in! Let yourself feel it. Feel it in your body – what are the sensations?

3. Write it down or make some other record of it. It's really helpful to have something tangible to look at during future difficult times.

HOW TO GET AFFIRMATIONS WORKING FOR YOU

An affirmation is a short, punchy, positive statement about yourself, your role in life, your values, character traits or something physical or emotional related to you. It's a statement that can become your mantra, supporting your core stability to keep you actively working within your own standards and capabilities. Affirmations remind your mind to sustain positivity throughout the day and encourage a full range of motion. They are the second half of your appreciation workout.

For some people, who have a good sense of their self-concept, a particular inclination towards positive thinking and a 'go-get-it' attitude, these short, punchy one-liners are super-helpful mindset reminders and don't require much extra effort.

If you are not that person, this can still work for you. In fact, all the more reason to explore the 'how' in this workout.

When I was working in addiction treatment centres, it was relatively common for clients to experience some form of relapse following affirmation work. To the untrained eye, this might seem odd because we are led to believe that affirmations make us feel better. I hope by explaining the process I will help you to understand that they target fundamental changes in how you feel about yourself and therefore may bring up difficult feelings.

Ultimately, if you're telling yourself 'I love me' when, in fact, you are living in a space of self-loathing, all that happens is that it feels incongruent and dishonest. If this is where you find yourself, you'll probably want to back up and tell me that affirmations don't work for you – you'll be sure that you are one of the very few who are not supposed to love life or enjoy self-care and, at the end of the day, looking after your psychological wellbeing is just not for you. I don't believe that for a second!

The thing we don't talk about often enough is that those one-liners I referred to above target just your frontal cortex (your thinking brain), and if you are dealing with a level of pain, trauma or disturbance that runs deeper than that – if you've got experiences that carry lots of shame – we have to get underneath your frontal cortex to figure out what you need and what's going to work for you. In this instance, using affirmations to look after your mental health needs to be slightly more forceful than it sounds on the surface; you can't just say the affirmation to yourself once or twice and expect your history and self-concept to shift into a positive mindset. If your mind is suffering with pain and shame and negative or limiting beliefs about yourself, the first step to retraining it is to flood it with positive affirmations, whether you believe them or not, and to go with the process, however incongruent it may at first feel.

Here are some examples for you to experiment with and see what reaction you have.

Pick any of the following affirmations or create your own, to be repeated to yourself three times per day:
- I am worth every ounce of the fight.
- I am safe to feel, heal and recover.
- I choose to love, cherish and accept myself, exactly as I am.
- I trust the timing of my life.
- I want to know myself.
- I am a success because I try.
- I live *now*.
- I am thankful.
- I am helpful.
- I accept my responsibility in life.

- I am vulnerable.
- I want to learn and grow.
- I can handle this.
- I am allowed to make mistakes.
- I am OK.
- I can be loved.
- I am capable of change.
- I am at peace.

(You can also use these to progress the stabilising thoughts (see p. 36) of your core-stability workout.)

Some technical pointers for creating your own affirmations

1. Affirmations are always written in the first person. That means no 'you', 'we', 'they' or 'us'.

2. They are always positive. For example, 'I am not ugly' is not an affirmation, whereas 'I am attractive' is.

3. They are also always done with compassion (a positive emotional charge) because they are challenging negative emotional charges (like shame and resentment). For example, an affirmation that challenges a shame-based belief about yourself such as 'I am useless' would need to be full of expansive compassion and sound something like: 'Today I am proud of the capable person I am becoming'.

4. Affirmations are ideally in the present tense but if that stirs up resistance, you can put them into future. For example – 'I am willing to have a happier, healthier mind' or 'I will have a happier, healthier mind'.

Now ask yourself: do I – or could I – believe these positive statements? If the answer is yes, you are already in good shape to integrate this workout into your daily routine. If the answer is no, let's have a look at something I call conversation affirmations.

The reason I developed conversation affirmations is because I spotted that many people can't identify with the one-liners on a long-term basis. They may start off working well, but then lose their power as time goes on, failing to heal what needs to be healed. Being able to expand the conversation around affirmations allows for more space and time for trial and error and, in so doing, it allows trust to be created between the different parts of you in question, thereby deepening your relationship with yourself.

JOURNAL OPPORTUNITY: CONVERSATION AFFIRMATIONS

To develop a personalised set of affirmations through exploring conversation affirmation for yourself, use your journal to consider how you felt when you were little, then as a teenager and as an adult. Did you feel safe? Did you feel you belonged? Did you feel allowed to be yourself? What did you need that you did not get?

As you consider the answers to these and any other questions that might organically arise from within you, start to develop the conversations you have with yourself. Listen carefully to what you needed historically and develop compassionate self-talk on the topics. You can write letters to different parts of yourself or simply speak out loud or in your mind. This is an exercise in exploration rather than a search for hard-and-fast answers. I would also suggest you take the conversations you are having to your therapeutic space, where possible.

Get affirmations working for you by reminding yourself that they are about protecting your self-concept. They work to defend your integrity and allow you to feel grounded, even when your outside world feels unsteady.

MENTAL HEALTH MYTH

'You have to love yourself wholeheartedly before you can love and be loved by others'

It's a nice idea that we need to find wholehearted self-love before we find another person who will love us the way we want and need to be loved. And the appreciation workout certainly moves us closer to self-love. But the truth is, if we have no idea how to love ourselves or there are parts of us that have never felt loved, how are you supposed to know what to do to demonstrate and feel a sense self-love? Sometimes we need to outsource our love in order to learn how to love ourselves). It's OK to look for love in others – the important thing is to explore how to internalise that love, rather than rely on the outsourcing to provide your love supply.

Your appreciation workout has been about changing, creating and protecting your self-concept and gratitude, and affirmations are how we got you there. Over time, this workout will bring contentment, peace and a happy glow into your life that is accessible on even your dullest and darkest days. You can take your appreciation workout anywhere with you. In fact, doing it in tandem with your mindfulness and connection workouts or while you are exercising will enhance its effect and leave you glowing inside and out.

This brings us towards the end of our programme and what we need now, as with any other workout, is a cooldown.

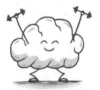 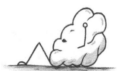 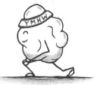

YOUR MENTAL HEALTH WORKOUT WEEKLY CHECKLIST

WEEKLY WORKOUTS	M	T	W	TH	F	S	SU
THERAPY							
SOCIAL EVENTS							
EXERCISE							
SELF-CARE							

DAILY WORKOUTS							
MINDFULNESS							
CONNECTION							
APPRECIATION							
MOVEMENT							

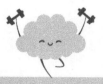

4 x Movement

As with any workout, the way we bring it all together is with a finisher (see previous chapter) and then a cooldown that will flush out the build-up of lactic acid and any unhelpful twinges to leave you feeling invigorated, empowered, motivated, happy and healthy.

This cooldown helps to release all the feelings you have been training with, pushing and pulling, bending and stretching. It rinses out any stiffness and brings you back to a place of balance. Balance and health are, of course, what we are aiming for.

So, your fourth and final daily mental health workout is, quite simply, movement.

MOVEMENT WORKOUT

1. Make a list of ways in which you can move. Make your bed, for example, or walk around the room you are in, stretch out your upper body, your lower body, go for a walk around the block, have a wiggle to your favourite song . . . Pretty much anything goes.

2. Check in with how the movement you do changes your feelings and thoughts on the inside.

3. Notice how energised and/or calm you feel physically.

4. Repeat x 4 per day.

WHY WE DO THIS WORKOUT

In the weekly workouts, we looked at how important formal exercise is for your mental health. Here, we are talking about moving your body naturally, which is an entirely separate thing. This is a great mental health workout for anyone who, for any reason, cannot or does not have the privilege of participating in formal exercise as described on pp. 106–8. (Yes, being able to exercise is indeed a luxury we don't always appreciate – you can put that on your gratitude list.)

How we move our bodies has a direct effect on our thoughts, feelings and behaviours. If I haven't made it clear enough yet, your mind, and therefore your mental health, doesn't just live in your brain – your mind is very much part of your body and this daily mental health workout helps you to use it to stay in touch with yourself as a whole.

In fact, often in therapy we draw attention to the movements made while someone is speaking. Movement can give us great insight into what's going on underneath the surface and is sometimes even more honest than what people are able to say. If we can tune in to our bodies, we can understand our mental health muscle better and be better able to hold on to that aligned, balanced, equal and worthy feeling we've been working on right from the start of this programme. Around 70 per cent of our communication is non-verbal, after all.

Feelings are energy in motion: e-motion (I did not come up with that, but I love it). Whether you are sitting still for long periods of time or working out in a structured way, your body still needs a chance to move naturally, organically and as it pleases. Formal exercise gets you fit and activates some helpful chemicals and muscle groups, as discussed; but ultimately, we have the option to engage with it or not. Natural movement is a non-negotiable for everyone; and everyone has a slightly different energy that moves in a slightly different way. Think about the mannerisms you recognise in the people you live and work closely with. This is a really good example of their unique way of moving. And you will have your own version – your own mannerisms and way of moving your body in a totally spontaneous and pure way.

As we go through our day-to-day experience, regardless of who we are and what we are doing, we consistently have emotional responses that we are both aware and unaware of. Natural movement provides the release our mental health muscle needs to keep it functioning healthily. You will notice when you put this book down that your body will do something natural: you might want to move and stretch, fall asleep, have a snack . . . These are all ways of your body processing some of the feelings that have been activated. If we don't move our bodies enough, those emotional responses turn into stagnant energy as the feelings languish inside us, and we risk these unprocessed emotions tuning into resentment and fear, then symptomatic issues like anxiety, stress and depression.

It is in this cooldown that we really and truly allow body and mind to come together and work with each other as one. The one tip I can give you here is to observe, observe, observe. What happens when you move? Do your feelings change? What happens to your thinking? Do different types of thoughts come in? If you move to different surroundings, how does that affect how you think and feel? What memories are activated? What are they telling you? How are you going to cope with those? You don't need to do anything with this information, just gather it and let it inform what you know about yourself.

Cast your mind back over everything you have learned about yourself and about psychology through Your Mental Health Workout journey and use this cooldown as an opportunity to assimilate that information, by applying it while moving. Instead of getting tied up with what others think when they look at you moving, or judging your body for how it moves, use your affirmations, say your gratitude list, do some mindfulness, call someone and connect while moving, it'll help to solidify your experience and create some muscle memory that both your body and mind can benefit from.

The other reason to move regularly is that it alerts you to any aches and pains that need attending to, both physically and emotionally. These will naturally be more noticeable the more mindful you are about yourself. For example – you may not realise you have a stiff neck until you try to move it. In addition, you can get feedback from others: use your social events and connection workouts to help with this. When you feel brave enough, ask your trusted people what *they* have observed about the way you move: do you walk slower or faster than most? Do you slouch when you are sad? You may like to use that information to inform how you do some of the other workouts in this book. For example, if you struggle with eye contact when you are angry, the next time you set a boundary with someone you are angry with, do your best to look them in the eye while doing it. You may also like to take what you notice to your therapeutic space, too.

Focusing on how you move throughout your day encourages new connections, insights, growth and ideas. We are not designed to be sitting still all day and we just learn better when moving is involved. While you've been reading through this programme, you'll have had hundreds and thousands of different internal reactions – most of them thoughts and feelings that have happened in your mind and sent signals to your body. While you are sitting still, those signals have nowhere to go and it is all too easy to get caught up in what is wrong with you, the things you do not understand and the anxieties and frustrations that cause you pain. Moving around on a regular basis allows your thoughts and feelings to do their thing, heightening your potential for positivity and your ability to connect with yourself, therefore benefiting all your other mental health workouts too.

HOW TO GET THIS WORKOUT WORKING FOR YOU

When I do workshops or group therapy I often talk about and include a movement section that allows people to simply walk around the room, seek out different movements stances and body language and notice the variations in thoughts, feelings and behaviours. Some people like this; others don't and find themselves feeling self-conscious.

Movement is particularly hard for those who have a negative body image or any other type of difficult relationship with their body. What research has shown us, however, is that imagining something happening can prepare your mind for doing exactly the thing you imagine. If movement is challenging for you for any reason, whether physical, physiological or psychological, try these mobilising visualisations to get you started:

1. On your own: imagine yourself doing a movement (particularly if self-consciousness is your issue, try to imagine doing it in the presence of others). By using your imagination, you get to explore and control exactly what happens with your body without judgment.

2. With other people: observe how others move around. In your brain you have things called mirror neurons acting as unconscious mimics; in essence, they fire off each time you see someone else move (this is partly why yawns are so contagious). By intentionally observing others, you start to exercise the same part of your mind as you would if you were also moving. Let your own form of physical movement develop over time.

The previous three workouts were a pretty in-depth exploration of your inside experiences, activating your mind in as many ways as possible and creating definition around your self-concept, as well as how you define yourself to others. Before that, in the weekly workout section, you activated all the major muscle groups that keep your mind strong and steady. This movement workout, being a cooldown, doesn't take as much effort as the rest for exactly that reason, but it is mighty in its results. Daily movement allows things to click into place that might not have already, because you feel it with your body, as well as your mind. We have spent plenty of time understanding how to realign ourselves and when that realignment happens, you'll know.

YOUR MENTAL HEALTH WORKOUT WEEKLY CHECKLIST

WEEKLY WORKOUTS	M	T	W	TH	F	S	SU
THERAPY							
SOCIAL EVENTS							
EXERCISE							
SELF-CARE							

DAILY WORKOUTS							
MINDFULNESS							
CONNECTION							
APPRECIATION							
MOVEMENT							

Chapter 6

A FINAL WORD

IF THIS WERE a physical workout, we would all be stretching out, wiping away the sweat on our foreheads and clapping right now.

Some of you might feel super-motivated, accomplished and proud of yourselves; others might be giving yourself a hard time over the bits that haven't gone as you wanted, or those you don't fully understand yet. This programme has laid the groundwork. It is now up to you to apply it and make it work for you, creating a world full of new opportunities for yourself. Your commitment to yourself makes you part of the generation that busts the stigma around mental health!

Part of the reason why I love my work as a therapist, mental health consultant and now also an author, is that what we can find out about our minds is never-ending; if you can maintain a level of curiosity and practise asking for help when you need it, this journey just continues to unravel. I have been in consistent therapy since the age of eighteen, and one thing I can tell you for sure is that I am still finding out about myself, working on myself and developing helpful ways of navigating this world. What does change over time, however, is that the effort involved moves from challenging and difficult to enjoyable, the more you do it. Just as if your body is getting used to a new form of movement, feeling sore to start off with, you need to give your mind the same chance.

That soreness means you might not feel better immediately, and sometimes you'll become aware of pain you didn't even know you had before starting these workouts. But trust yourself – your courage is more powerful than your pain. In the same way that there are marks and scars on your body, the wounds and breaks in your soul create an individual trademark that only you have the authority to work with.

As you go forward in your life, the workouts presented here will support you to figure yourself out and design a life you are excited to live. As at the start of the programme, my suggestion is that you apply all the workouts for five weeks and see which work best for you – then, in week six, you can decide what you would like to integrate into your life and what you would prefer to leave behind for now (you can always come back and get it if you change your mind).

The main difference I usually point out between mental and physical health is that to do a physical workout you can apply yourself for thirty to sixty minutes at a time (on average) and be done with it. Mental health needs to be approached as an ongoing lifestyle choice, and Your Mental Health Workout helps you to do just that. You must not become complacent.

Working on your mental health is a lifelong investment in yourself and it also contributes to wider change. Your

Mental Health Workout is just one stop on your journey. When you tune in with your thoughts, feelings and behaviours and then remove the judgments, criticisms and hate from your inside world, you remove them from your outside world, too. Imagine the world we would live in if everybody did that.

One of the saddest things about the stigma attached to mental health is that the longer it sticks around, the bigger the effect it has on our self-esteem and our ability to ask for help. If we go on allowing mental health to be defined as some kind of taboo, it will continue to be subject to discrimination. We live in a time when so much is changing – why leave mental wellbeing behind?

So, on the days when you feel depleted and unmotivated, remember this: if we all worked on our mental health in the same way we do our physical health, the world would be a much kinder, happier place. We would still experience conflict and trouble at times, but our capacity to cope with difficulty increases exponentially when we work on our minds in line with our bodies.

Each time you do a workout you will feel differently about it. There will be good days and bad. You will have slips, lapses and relapses and probably even give up altogether and restart a few times. The hard-and-fast rule is not to give yourself a hard time about anything that happens. It is all learning; it is all experience.

If you work on this programme in a pair or in a group, remember that Your Mental Health Workout looks different on everyone, so do not compare your insides to what you see on other people's outsides – it's simply not fair. You can, however, without judgment or comparison, look for the similarities and the things you can relate to – the ones that validate your experience. There will always be differences and opportunities to compare ourselves but it is the similarities that bring us together.

You are always free to modify your workout to support you and/or your mental state at any given time, and always remember that if something feels like too much for you at any moment, stop; go and work on something else, strengthening and stretching other areas of your mind, and then come back to the more difficult bits later. You will learn to challenge yourself to deal with feeling uncomfortable, but not to push yourself to the point of injury. Uncomfortable is where the change happens; pain is where the damage sets in. *This is about healing, not winning.*

A healthy mind is something everyone deserves – it's not a luxury – and by applying Your Mental Health Workout as a lifestyle choice, you have moved yourself closer to this basic human right. Your mind is precious: appreciate it. Love it. Work for it. It is the only one you are going to get.

APPENDICES

Appendix 1

PHYSIO FOR YOUR FEELINGS

THIS SECTION IS effectively optional because it sits separately to or alongside the 5-week programme, but I'd suggest you give it a glance, as it offers you something to dip in and out of at your leisure. You can also add these exercises to the main weekly and daily ones to create individualised progressions within Your Mental Health Workout.

Physiotherapy is usually understood as supporting recovery of movement and function when we are physically injured. It can also help to reduce the risk of injury in the future. Your mind needs something similar when going through change. We've talked a lot about feelings throughout this programme and worked with them extensively. Even so, they are difficult, and sometimes feeling your feelings can feel like a bit too much. So in this chapter you will find a range of 'physio' exercises you can apply to specific feelings, as and when they come up.

The way to use this section is to refer to it when you notice a particular feeling is causing you to feel overwhelmed or is coming up more frequently and with more intensity than you would like. Once again, we are not trying to take away your feelings here; rather, I am providing you with tools to build faith in yourself to know exactly how to feel your feelings, what to do with them and enable you to have a happier experience.

Use them when you become aware of a limitation in your progress and want to feel better supported in a particular area, or simply because you find yourself a bit overwhelmed and need something different to work with. You can also use them if you feel out of your depth at any point in the programme or if you become aware of particular psychological injuries along the way.

These workouts are specific and targeted, but they also consider your mind as a whole, so you'll notice lots of cross-overs with both the main workout and within these more targeted ones which, hopefully, will make them easier to apply.

Feeling your Feelings

I am aware that it is very easy for me to tell you to 'feel your feelings'. Yet it is quite a difficult thing to do. Here are some steps to get you started with the 'feelings physio'.

 TO FEEL YOUR FEELINGS PHYSIO EXERCISE

- Identify the signals and sensations in your body – for example, tension in your shoulders, cold feet, a heavy or light feeling in your stomach.

- Name the feeling if you can, or find three words to describe it.
- Observe if and how the signals and sensations change as you acknowledge them.
- Ask yourself what message this feeling gives you.
- Fully acknowledge it.
- Express gratitude towards your feelings for guiding you to a better understanding of your mental health and emotional wellbeing.

Following this, you'll probably be asking: 'Now, what do I do with those feelings I've just spent time feeling?'

WHAT TO DO WITH THE FEELINGS PHYSIO EXERCISE

- Understand that your feelings are your mental health muscle; they are important and valid and give you information about what you need to do next.
- Identify whether the action you need to take is internal or external, visible or invisible.
- If it is an internal or invisible movement, use a self-soothing technique, such as something from your external self-care kit (see p. 121), to support and build your emotional resilience.
- If it is visible to others, i.e. it is happening externally, reflect on what behaviour is going to be the most compassionate choice for you.

Clearing Emotional Blockages

Despite feeling your feelings and knowing what to do with them, things can sometimes get blocked – particularly if your thoughts and feelings are a bit muddled. The muddle is sometimes called an 'emotional blockage', and here are some steps to help you release it. You can use this at any point during the programme if you feel stuck. Sometimes a blockage is not conscious, but we can still become aware of it if we give ourselves the space and time in which to do so. Therefore, it's worth using this physio exercise as a self-check-in from time to time too.

1. Listen in to your body and mind (you can use your mindful hold – see p. 133). Identify the thought or feeling that is getting in the way.

2. Say it out loud to yourself.

3. What is your reaction to saying that to yourself?

4. Say the exact opposite to yourself.

5. What is your reaction to saying the opposite to yourself?

6. Which do you prefer?

7. Repeat.

The following physio exercises target specific feelings. Applying these will give you more authority over the intensity with which you exercise your feelings.

Joy

Let me start this one by saying that in the main, most people don't complain about feeling too happy or having too much joy in their lives. But when we are happy and joyful, it is important to know how to harness that so that we can avoid the fear of losing it, as if it will be taken away from us. Here are some steps you can take to allow yourself to fully experience your joy and maintain a base level of happiness.

1. Seek balance in all areas.

2. Know that happiness is contagious; it breeds success and allows you to reap the rewards.

3. Write down in a creative way all the things that make you happy. In 2015, I wrote down on Post-it notes all the things that made me happy throughout the year and put them in a jar. At the end of the year, I emptied the jar and read through them all. Despite the usual ups and downs, I had no excuse but to smile at the happy moments I'd reflected on throughout the year.

Love

Love is one of the most universal experiences and I talk about it *a lot* as something that heals us. Loving others and loving ourselves, as well as being loved and knowing how to let love in – even to the parts of us that have never been loved – is an ever-emerging and restorative process. Here are some ideas on practising letting love in:

- Make sure you are listening for the love messages coming your way – the compliments, the kind acts, the observations and the quality time.
- Add the love messages you have given or received to your gratitude list and use them to form your affirmations.
- Before you ignore or reject them, say 'thank you' to the other person, or at least have a moment of internal acknowledgment that they happened.
- When it comes to acts of love, remember to hold on to the moment and create a memory, rather than using them to build future expectations which can lead to disappointment and, ultimately, resentment.
- Consider that you are loveable just as you are, and that you are just as entitled to love and be loved as anyone else.
- Remember that love changes.
- Remember that someone's inability to love you is not a reflection of your worth as a person.

Anger

You are highly likely to experience anger at some point during the programme, and in life in general – and that is a good thing. Anger only gets in our way when we don't know how to use it for good. Be curious about it, rather than trying to hide it. Ask yourself the following questions:

- What have you learned about anger in your life?
- Is it inappropriate?
- Unreasonable?
- Unattractive?
- Unsafe?
- How did the people in your family get angry? Were they passive-aggressive (expressing their anger indirectly through silent treatment and being sarcastic) or were they ragers? Or somewhere in between?
- Did you grow up fearing anger? And/or do your best to avoid it?

Despite the negative connotations sometimes attached to anger, it is natural, and it is necessary. It alerts us to danger and empowers us to take action. It informs our boundaries and allows us to see our worth. When we deny our anger, we fog up our souls, damage our hearts and renounce our truth. Anger is much closer to love than we are led to believe: without anger, we cannot love fully. Let anger be part of your journey.

1. Stop and count to ten. This gives your thoughts and feelings time to catch up with each other and re-coordinate themselves if you have become dysregulated.

2. Become willing to work on your anger. When you become willing, you will start to feel less resistance and you will take the charge out of your angry feelings. From this place it becomes possible to go near them.

3. Recognise the impact of anger on your body. Stay interested in the impact on you and you will become aware of the impact your anger could have on others.

4. Take a moment to respect the emotion by allowing it to give you a message. Mostly, the message we get here is that we are not OK with something and that what is happening causes us to feel scared and threatened.

5. Use the energy anger gives you to motivate you, and respect your anger by setting boundaries in response to it. Used well, anger can power you up and inspire you to make healthy changes to your world.

Note: anger often interacts with other emotions, particularly fear; sometimes it can feel easier to be angry than fearful, sad, vulnerable and powerless. Know that you are probably going to experience some fear, too, and use the fear workout on p. 208 to help you understand anything fear-related that comes up.

Pain

If your pain was physical, you would probably not be able to ignore it for any length of time. We can all do ourselves a favour by thinking about emotional pain as we would physical and tending to it in a similar way.

1. Acknowledge the type of pain you are in. Is it sadness, loneliness, grief, etc.?

2. Approach the feelings; do not avoid them. Use the physio exercises in this section to ensure your pain gets the attention it needs. For example, if you feel sad or if you feel shame, follow the relevant suggested steps. Remaining interested and curious about what is going on, without judgment, is the best psychological-pain-management tool.

3. Do things that make you feel competent and comfortable (AKA self-soothing). If it was physical pain, you'd take the pressure off for a bit while you heal – that doesn't mean the pain goes away, but you can self-soothe throughout to make it more manageable.

4. Try to stay away from self-medicating – i.e. drugs, alcohol, eating on your feelings, overworking, overexercising and things like people-pleasing. Self-medicating in these ways only robs you of the opportunity to work with your feelings. Instead, work

to build emotional tolerance and learn from what is happening in your feelings and thoughts.

Shame

We all have an experience of shame at some point. In part, healthy shame (if we can call it that) helps us to behave well in social situations. For example, we wear clothes because going outside naked would be considered quite shameless in most cultures (but not all, might I point out). Shame ensures you adhere to the social constructs around you, and that can be helpful because it keeps you safe; but it can also be desperately unhelpful at times because it creates the narrative that your worth is based on society and culture, rather than your individual drives and desires. So we need to be able to navigate shame and find our way out of it. The main antidotes are compassion and observation. Shame wants us to hide away and to keep secrets, but if we do so, our darkness and unhappiness can pull us away from our mental health goals. It breeds and can lead to a miserable experience of always feeling less than others and worthless. So, it is vital that you find a safe space to expose it. Try the following:

1. Acknowledge the physical response in your body. If it is not safe to do this in the situation that you feel ashamed in, do it in hindsight. Are you (or were you) hot, cold, shaking, frozen, for example?

2. Name this physical response as shame. (At this point, please try not to buy into feeling ashamed of shame – it's not very helpful.) Literally say to yourself: 'I am feeling shame right now and I need to remind myself that I am still good enough, worthy enough as a human being'. You could use one of your affirmations on repeat here to really tackle it head-on.

3. When you feel able, talk to your therapist, counsellor, mental health professional or trusted other. Or you can brain purge in your journal about the experience that you are having. Do these things not because they can take the feeling away, but because shame dies (or at least lessens) on exposure.

4. Challenge the desire to hide away when you feel the shame rise by looking your therapist or trusted other in the eye. Or, if you wrote in your journal, read the passage back to yourself a few days later and answer it as if you were responding to someone you love . . . what would you say?

5. Notice the intensity lessening.

Fear

People often ask me how they can be more brave or coura-geous, take more risks in life or be more spontaneous? The answer is always: work *with* your fear, rather than against it.

Courage is not the absence of fear. It is the action of feeling fear and leaning into it instead of running away.

Give this a shot if you are working with fear:

1. Pay attention to your fear, rather than trying to avoid it and pretending you are not fearful. Create the willingness to do something differently and activate your courage.

2. Notice your fearful thinking and ask yourself what it is that you are really frightened of right now. Write it down as a way of externalising it.

3. Resist the urge to stay where you are and let the fear control you. Change happens when we feel uncomfortable, so allow yourself to feel uncomfortable.

4. Hold it! Stay with the tension between wanting to go back to what you know and challenging yourself. Work with the feelings and thoughts that come up to create psychological strength and resilience.

5. Repeat as necessary.

Guilt

The difference between shame and guilt is that shame tells us we are 'wrong' and 'worthless' as a whole, whereas guilt informs us that we have done something wrong.

I have also seen people use guilt as a kind of defence against feeling out of control, disrespected and angry. It can feel easier to tell ourselves that we have done something wrong and we have to fix it than to stand up for ourselves and set boundaries with others. Guilt can also come up during the bargaining phase of grief, as a way of trying to gain control over a narrative that we cannot change.

Explore your guilty feelings. Find space and time to ask yourself the following questions (write down the answers in your journal if it helps):

- Why do I feel guilt?
- What part of me does it come from?
- Is there anything to gain by feeling guilty?
- Does it hold me back?
- Is it reasonable?

Try this to help you navigate guilt:

1. Write down the story you are telling yourself. Mostly, guilt functions to regulate us. And sometimes we take that a bit far and try to use it to regulate or influence things that are outside of our control. The story you tell yourself – 'I should have done it differently', 'It is my fault because . . .' – is, in part, your mind's attempt to regain some mastery over the situation, which, in reality, is not possible.

2. Make amends by saying sorry if you have hurt someone in any way. Words are fine, but actions are

usually better, so also commit to changing your behaviour going forward. In my opinion, that is the real apology. The big thing here is that it is not about the other person and how they respond; it is about you hearing yourself and seeing yourself doing something differently.

3. Forgive. Find compassion and understanding for yourself. We usually manage to hurt others by mistake, because we didn't know any different or lacked the appropriate tools to deal with a situation. It is only when we forgive ourselves that we can really receive and accept forgiveness from others.

Stress

Our minds are always aiming for balance. When we feel 'stressed', we have become aware that we have been off balance for some time. Although Your Mental Health Workout is a stress-management tool in general, it is important you also know what to do in those moments you feel stressed and simply need to regain a feeling of balance before continuing.

1. Permission: Give yourself permission to step away from the thing that is stressing you out. No excuses, step back. This is the equivalent of allowing the swelling to come down with a physical injury.

2. Exercise: Gently get the balance of cortisol and adrenaline where it needs to be through movement. During a stressful time, exercise can have immediately positive effects. It helps calm the nervous system.

3. Connection: Heal the injury through talking to others. Most stress responses stem from an emotionally charged place. Connection takes the charge out and encourages healing. (See pp. 148–151 for more on connection.)

4. Plan and programme: Make a plan to help you feel safe and make any difficult decisions, preferably while you are in a calm and balanced state of mind – but the act of planning can also help calm your nervous system, so do it whenever you feel ready.

Letting Go

Letting go is not a feeling, strictly speaking. It is an emotional experience and can be hard because we'd usually rather live with the pain we recognise than face something unfamiliar.

People who are genuinely able let go have been practising it for years – trust me! And even then, things can be difficult. But it is definitely worth some extra attention, and you can start the process now by applying the physio below.

1. Become *conscious* of what you are holding on to that no longer serves you. Get present and become aware of

reliving your past. Make the conscious choice to let it go.

2. *Commit* yourself to working on letting go. This is an active decision, not a passive one. It involves you working to stay aligned with what you need to do, and you only need your own permission to let go – no one else's. This sometimes involves forgiveness.

3. *Communicate* and express the pain and hurt that you feel. If you can, represent yourself and hear yourself speaking your truth.

4. *Cease* being the victim and blaming others. Take responsibility for your own happiness. Don't give the person who hurt you so much power.

5. Believe that *change* is possible.

Rejection

Again, strictly speaking this is not a feeling. But, when we have an experience of rejection we are likely to feel shame and pain, and when we are in that place, our core stability suffers and we find it a challenge to set boundaries, as we become too vulnerable.

We have all felt 'rejected' at some point, and therefore we all have varying levels of 'rejection sensitivity'. It is important to remember that rejection can be both obvious and subtle, and interestingly, when we feel emotionally or, indeed, phys-ically rejected, we experience a somatic pain, which means it happens in our bodies as well as our minds. With that in mind, I am sure some physio will not go amiss.

Rejection often starts in a social context and may not be about you, but the person doing the rejecting. In response, as an attempt at not feeling the pain of rejection we start to reject ourselves and learn to expect rejection from others. So, this physio exercise is about you not rejecting yourself.

1. Assess your level of rejection sensitivity: how sensitive do you think you are to rejection right now?

2. Find the root of the rejection sensitivity: think back to the first time you can remember feeling rejected – what happened?

3. Invite those feelings in by acknowledging the pain, the shame, the anger, etc. It is likely that this memory is painful and sad, and therefore you have put effort into not feeling or remembering this root cause, so rejecting yourself.

Work on not rejecting yourself by using your feelings to inform you of what you need:

- If you feel sad, what do you need?
- If you feel angry, what do you need?
- If you feel shame, what do you need?
  (Use the other feeling physio exercises to help you here.)

4. Use the self-connection and mindfulness workouts in the main programme (see pp. 134 and 149) to integrate this into your life.

Letting Go of Control

We control things because we believe that this will change how we feel on the inside. It is a dangerous place to be – relying on outside entities to dictate our mental health – and it leads to internal and, eventually, external chaos, causing poor mental health and, ultimately social disharmony.

Use this physio exercise to release yourself from the trap that is control, to embrace your vulnerability and allow change to occur. You will gain empowerment over the things you *can* control by recognising those you cannot.

1. Acknowledge that you, alone, cannot control anything outside of yourself. You are likely to feel helpless and powerless.

2. Write down your fears. Be honest. You can come back to this time and time again. Our fears change depending on how honest we can be, and control thrives off fear. Each time you check in with yourself, you can also do a check-in with how your fears have evolved, changed and developed.

3. Ask for help: share the fears you wrote down with a trusted other. Connection is key. If you stay in social

isolation and make no effort to share with others, you will indeed feel you can control your own bubble. The danger is that at some point, inevitably, you will be proved wrong, and you want your landing to be as soft as possible. Asking for help and sharing your fears is a really good sign of recovery and contributes to reconnecting with others.

4. Feel the pain. We change when we see the light, but we also change when we feel the pain. This works in tandem with your boundary and vulnerability workout (see p. 48).

5. Reinforce helpful external factors, while remembering that you cannot influence them directly: look for people, places and things that you can rely on but do not depend on to define your mood or actions – for example, a close friend who knows you well, your favourite safe space (bedroom, coffee shop, gym) or maybe you have a cherished item or object that helps you to feel safe in your letting-go experience.

Hope

Hope is something we are attempting to cultivate throughout Your Mental Health Workout. Some of us are naturally more hopeful than others, but there are ways you can actively bring some more hope into your life:

1. Look for hope in others. Have people around you in whom you can see hope.

2. Seek out creative solutions. Think outside the box when it comes to problem solving.

3. Challenge your negative thinking. Use your appreciation workout to help you here (see p. 170).

4. Do the stuff you love. Be active in bringing love, joy and happiness into your lifestyle.

5. Be brave.

6. Be kind.

Appendix 2

MODIFICATIONS AND
PROGRESSIONS

— — — —

THE MODIFICATIONS IN this chapter are simple changes you can make to accommodate specific identifiable mental health needs. You can also use them as progressive additions to the main 5-week programme. They are not a substitute for evidence-based treatments like medication and therapy; they are simply basic steps for you to take in order to look after yourself throughout Your Mental Health Workout. These basic workouts will not heal all your mental health challenges, but they might just make a little bit of difference when you need it most.

It's worth reading through the following in case there is something here that you can identify with and find helpful. You will notice many crossovers with the main workout. It is likely that at some point in our lives, we will all experience some form of anxiety, obsession, depression and self-sabotage, and what I want you to gain by reading this section is a better understanding of how you can target specific symptoms when they arise.

Generalised or Specific
Feelings of Anxiety

Most of us will feel anxious at some point in our lives. For some, anxiety is very specific, while for others, it is more general.

Generalised anxiety can be attached to a wide range of issues. Sufferers often find it very hard to relax. If you worry about a multitude of things or, indeed, seek out reasons to be anxious, you might like to try this workout on a daily basis.

These steps will also work for anyone who experiences anxiety in response to specific situations, circumstances or events.

1. Self-soothe: this is where your external self-care is really useful (see p. 120). Do things that will make you feel nice and calm your nervous system. It gets you out of your fight-flight-freeze trauma response.

2. Connect and share with others: anxieties often feel a lot bigger when they stay in your head. Rumination breeds rumination. Speak it out.

3. Face feelings: the word 'anxiety' is usually used to describe a build-up of feelings that have overwhelmed your mind. When the mind is too full, the body takes over and you'll start to get those anxious sensations in your voluntary muscles, like an urge to pace, twitchy

hands and feet and feeling that you need to stay very still or move about a lot. If your anxiety is more chronic, you might also experience changes in your involuntary muscle groups (or striated muscles) in the form of a racing heart, palpitations, breathlessness or a sudden urge to use the toilet. Once you have self-soothed any physical sensations and taken the power out of the anxiety through connection, become curious about the feelings involved in creating it. Fear and anger are usually the main players, in my experience.

4. Focus on what you *can* change: often, when we are anxious, we worry and obsess about stuff that will never happen or things we cannot change. Find something in your life that you *do* have control over – something you *can* change and focus on that. This needs to be about you; you can't change other people, places or things.

Note: this is not a one-time thing – you will need to work on these steps consistently, over a period of time, in order to see a reduction in anxious responses.

Social Anxiety

People who have social anxiety can come across as shy and therefore be labelled as introverted, allowing painful experiences of social anxiety to slide under the radar. (See also p. 94.) Social anxiety is far more than feeling shy though; it is an intense experience of fear and panic over day-to-day activities that involve socialising. Most of us worry about social situations on some level, but someone who has social anxiety feels as if they might be publicly humiliated or embarrassed to the extent that any social interaction, or even the thought of one, can trigger an anxious response in the body. The response might be low-level blushing or starting to sweat or it could be a full-on anxiety attack in which the person is so overloaded with fear that their mind thinks they are in imminent danger and they need to fight, flee or freeze. With social anxiety, the worry does not pass once you have evidence that you are safe, so you have to find ways to self-soothe during social events, so that the worry before, during and after doesn't immobilise you.

1. Self-soothe: make a list of internal and external activities that help your nervous system feel calm.

2. Connect: anxiety feels a lot bigger when we leave it to fester in our minds. Connect with one person you feel safe around.

3. Feelings: once you've self-soothed and connected with someone else, take a moment to acknowledge the feelings that contributed to you feeling socially anxious. Fear, panic and anger are usually the main players (see the foundation feelings chart on pp. 14–5 for help with this).

4. Focus on the things you can control: whether it is your breath, your schedule, how you move your body and,

eventually, your thoughts and feelings (when they've calmed down enough for you to connect with them).

5. Repeat as necessary.

Adjustments for Coping with Obsessions and Compulsions

Lots of us experience obsessions and compulsions in one or more areas of our lives.

Obsessions are unwanted thoughts that preoccupy you. Compulsions are a feeling that you *have* to behave in a certain way, as if you have no other option. Frequently, they are just our minds' way of trying to make sense of stuff that feels quite messy. For example, if you are in a relationship that is a bit all over the place emotionally, or you are going through something difficult like grief, obsessions and compulsions can develop as a way to contain the metaphorical messiness of what you are experiencing. However, sometimes they become so severe that they turn into addictions or obsessive-compulsive disorders. Ultimately, they are driven by our anxiety, which is built on feelings.

Lots of Your Mental Health Workout is about you feeling empowered and gaining choice and authority over your life. Obsessions and compulsions need a specific type of attention in order to be within our authority. If they are severe enough to warrant a diagnosis of OCD or addiction in any form, help from a specialist is the way to go, but in the meantime, you can consider the following steps:

1. Sit up. Pay attention and activate your courage.

2. Pull up your fearful thoughts, doubts and situations –
   i.e. think about the thoughts that trigger the obsessions
   or compulsions.

3. Push back. Resist the urge to act out on your
   compulsions.

4. Hold it! Stay with the tension between the obsession
   and the compulsion by acknowledging the obsession
   and not acting on the compulsive urge.

As an example that anyone can try, next time you want to
pick up your phone because you got a notification or you're
just about to scroll through messages and social media (an
obsession many of us have) – wait a few extra moments.
That tension you feel in between the obsession and the
compulsion (to pick the phone up) is where you need to be
working in order to reduce the power of both and to build
strength and range of motion in this area. Do something
self-soothing instead.

5. Repeat. Throughout Your Mental Health Workout,
   do these steps each time you feel an obsession or a
   compulsion pulling you away from your mental health
   goals.

Depression

Reactive or neurotic depression is the term we use to describe the experience of a low mood that has a negative effect on your wellbeing more than half the time. Organic or psychotic depression, the type that comes from a chemical imbalance, often needs medication (dependent on approach) and careful monitoring by yourself and at least one professional. There are some really basic things you can do to help yourself when you feel able in the meantime, if you feel you have either reactive or organic depression.

- Stay connected to others.
- Exercise regularly.
- Use a bright light therapy lamp for thirty minutes a day or get thirty minutes' worth of natural sunlight.
- Plan your activities each day, even if it's just the time you will get up and have a shower. Stick to it and build it each week.

Reality Checking for Those Recovering From Trauma

Reality checking is a really simple type of mental health physio we can all do with from time to time, especially when it comes to identifying trauma reactions.

Reality checking calls for fluid and accurate movement of your mental health muscle. Along with your mindfulness workout, it is a way of ensuring that you are present and working with what is happening right now, while checking to see if the stress, anxiety, trauma or pain you feel are, in fact, related to historic injuries or the present moment.

1. What thoughts are you having right now?

2. What is happening in front of you right now?

3. Do they match each other and make sense?

4. If so, you have a good handle on your reality; if not, you are likely to be experiencing a thinking distortion or cognitive pull, as we have called them (see p. 140), based in a trauma reaction.

If the latter is the case:

- Look around and name five things you can see right now to bring you into the present reality.
- Focus on your breath.
- Connect with others; refer to the connection workout on p. 149 to explore how connection heals trauma.

Self-sabotage

We can self-sabotage through addiction, an eating disorder, people-pleasing, perfectionism or any number of ways. I talked about self-medication briefly earlier (see p. 205), and that too can be a form of self-sabotage. Here are some steps you can take to get past the saboteur inside you:

1. **Identify *what* you are sabotaging.** You might already have this in the bag, but it's important to know what exactly it is you are sabotaging so that you can tell when you've made the changes. Try not to generalise about your life here – get really specific.

2. **Notice *how* you sabotage yourself.** There are so many ways we can sabotage ourselves. Get really mindful here and interested in how you do it. And again, be specific.

3. **Figure out *when* you are most likely to do it.** Trust me, it's not random. There will be a pattern – a particular way, a specific trigger and model for your sabotage. When it happens, get really interested in what takes place just before, then see what you can notice about your saboteur patterns.

4. **Ask yourself what it would be like to do things differently.** You don't have to find a way to change it right now (the appreciation workout on p. 170 will help you with that) – just start with asking the question, get that part of your brain mobilised and see what happens next.

SUGGESTED FURTHER READING

THE FOLLOWING IS a list of other authors, psychotherapists and influencers who have contributed to my training, learning and the development of Your Mental Health Workout. Although none of them is quoted directly in this book, these experts have had a significant impact and input in my professional training over the years.

Below are their names, along with some suggestions for further reading. However, many have a much wider range of books you can choose from.

Aaron Beck – American psychiatrist considered to be the father of cognitive behavioural therapy (CBT):
   Cognitive Therapy of Depression, 1978
   Cognitive Therapy and the Emotional Disorders, 1976
   Cognitive Therapy of Substance Abuse, 1977
   Anxiety Disorders and Phobias, 1985
   Love is never Enough, 1988

Carl Rogers – American psychologist who was among the founders of our widely regarded person-centred and humanistic approach to psychology:

On Becoming a Person, 1956

Freedom to Learn, 1968

Active Listening, 1957

Pia Mellody – one of the pioneers in treating co-dependency and relational trauma through looking at the childhood origins of emotional dysfunction. I was lucky enough to be trained in her trauma reduction model and continue to use parts of her approach within my clinical work:

Facing Codependence, 1989

Facing Love Addiction, 1992

The Intimacy Factor, 2003

Em Farrell – supervised my work for over five years and has been fundamental to me in gaining the compassion and confidence I hold within both my clinical work and my writing. She is a psychotherapist and supervisor in her own right too:

Lost for words, 1995

A is for Anorexia, 2015

Tian Dayton – psychologist, author and psychodramatist known for her work on 'emotional sobriety' with children of addicts and alcoholics:

The ACOA Trauma Syndrome, 2012

Trauma and Addiction, 2000

Emotional Sobriety, 2007

Gabor Maté – physician with a special interest in childhood development and trauma:
    Hold on to Your Kids, 2004
    Scattered Minds, 1999
    When the Body Says No, 2003
    In the Realm of Hungry Ghosts, 2008

Bessel van der Kolk – author, researcher and educator who focuses on the causes and effects of post-traumatic stress disorder:
    The Body Keeps the Score, 2014
    Traumatic Stress (ed.), 1996
    Psychological Trauma, 1987

Melody Beattie – author, known for her work on co-dependence and setting boundaries in particular:
    Codependent No More, 1986
    The Language of Letting Go, 1990
    Beyond Codependency, 1989

Brené Brown – researcher of shame and vulnerability. Brené is known for her books, lectures and podcast in recent years.
    Daring Greatly, 2012
    Dare to Lead, 2018
    The Gifts of Imperfection, 2010
    Rising Strong, 2015

John Bowlby – British psychologist, psychiatrist and psycho-analyst known for his interest in attachment and childhood development:

A Secure Base, 1988

Separation, 1972

Attachment and Loss (volumes 1, 2 and 3), 1969–80

The Making and Breaking of Affectional Bonds, 1979

Mary Ainsworth – American psychologist known for her work on attachment theory; often worked with John Bowlby (above):

Patterns of Attachment, 1978

Marsha M. Linehan – American psychologist and author; she created dialectical behavioural therapy (DBT), which is now widely used in a number of mental health treatments:

Cognitive Behavioral Treatment of Borderline Personality Disorder, 1983

DBT Skills Training Manual, 2014

Building a Life Worth Living, 2020

John Lee – pioneer in the therapeutic fields of anger, co-dependency, creativity, relationships and men's issues:

The Flying Boy, 1987

Facing the Fire, 1993

Writing from the Body, 1994

Growing Yourself Back Up, 2001

ADDITIONAL SUPPORT

Alternative Therapeutic Spaces

In this book, we talked about finding a therapeutic space that works for you. Here are some options for you to consider:

Find a one-to-one therapist who can see you on a weekly basis. If you feel comfortable doing so, ask around and see if you can get a name through word of mouth. Otherwise, you can search the following websites (UK-based):

- www.psychologytoday.com
- www.psychotherapy.org.uk
- bacp.co.uk
- www.counselling-directory.org.uk

You can find low-cost therapy through the following organisations:

- thebowlbycentre.org.uk
- spiralcentre.org
- freepsychotherapynetwork.com/organisations-offering-low-cost-psychotherapy/

If you would like to try out a group setting, there are a number of focused free or low-cost support groups available worldwide. Here are the UK websites, but there will be a version of these available in most countries:

Alcoholics Anonymous – www.alcoholics-anonymous.org.uk
Narcotics Anonymous – ukna.org
Overeaters Anonymous – www.oagb.org.uk
Co-dependents Anonymous – coda.org
Sex and Love Addiction Anonymous – www.slaauk.org
Anorexics and Bulimics Anonymous – aba12steps.org
Gamblers Anonymous – www.gamblersanonymous.org.uk
Debtors Anonymous – debtorsanonymous.org.uk
Workaholics Anonymous – workaholics-anonymous.org
Underearners Anonymous – www.underearnersanonymous.org
Adult Children of Alcoholics Anonymous –
    www.adultchildrenofalcoholics.co.uk

As their names suggest, these are a network of anonymous twelve-step groups that tackle specific issues. If any of these is of interest to you, check out their website and even go along to a meeting if you feel up to it. Understand that walking into a room full of new people can be terrifying, but the programme and support they offer is well worth facing your fears.

Further Resources

In addition to all of the above, for further support you can visit my website at www.zoeaston.com or www.yourmental-healthworkout.com

And here are some other websites and phone numbers if you find yourself needing immediate help:

MIND
www.mind.org.uk
0300 1233393

BRITISH ASSOCIATION FOR COUNSELLING AND PSYCHOTHERAPY
www.bacp.co.uk

UK COUNCIL FOR PSYCHOTHERAPY
www.psychotherapy.org.uk

SAMARITANS
www.samaritans.org
116 123

YOUNG MINDS
youngminds.org.uk
0808 802 5544

RETHINK
www.rethink.org
0300 5000 927

ACTION ON ADDICTION
www.actiononaddiction.org.uk
0300 330 0659

SHOUT – CRISIS TEXT LINE
Text 'SHOUT' to 85258
– in a mental health emergency

PAPYRUS UK
www.papyrus-uk.org
0800 068 4141
Text line – 07860 039967

CAMPAIGN AGAINST LIVING MISERABLY (CALM)
www.thecalmzone.net
0800 585858

SANE
www.sane.org.uk
07984 967708

NHS MENTAL HEALTH SERVICES
www.nhs.uk/conditions/stress-anxiety-depression/free-therapy-or-counselling/
Call – 111

You can also visit www.helplines.org for a wider list of mental health helplines.

ACKNOWLEDGEMENTS

IT IS SAFE to say that hundreds of people have provided me with the critical information and experience used to put this programme and book together – clients, therapists, friends, family and social media followers.

I want to say a particular thank you to Adela who was my therapist for over a decade and supported me throughout my recovery from trauma, my eating disorder and self-harming. And also Annemarie, who sat with me for months while I was in treatment, chipping away at what needed to be done to save my life.

Of course, as my supervisor, Em Farrell has been funda-mental to my emotional support throughout the writing of this book, not to mention the indispensable knowledge and skills she has passed on to me.

I'd also like to thank my agent, Ben Clark, the team of people at Yellow Kite books – in particular, Carolyn Thorne for believing in my idea and supporting me along the way with nothing but interest and compassion – and also Anne Newman, who asked all the right questions at the right time and got my message to a place where it is readable, digestible and helpful.

Of course, my lovely family deserve a huge thank you. Thank you to my mum, dad, sister and partner, who have witnessed this process and listened to me yo-yo through the various creative stages of horrendous self-doubt and then enhanced self-belief.

Last but not least, thank you to my readers and social media followers who have been invaluable in helping me to make working on mental health as accessible and acceptable as working on physical health.

INDEX

ABOUT THE AUTHOR

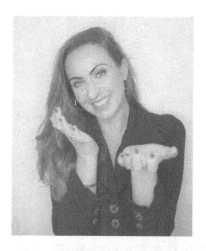

Photograph by Amber Pollack

Zoë Aston is a London-based psychotherapist and mental health consultant. With over a decade of therapeutic experience from her personal life and professional endeavours, she now brings therapy out of the therapeutic space to a mass audience to make support available to all who want it. She runs a private psychotherapy practice and works as a mental health consultant for boutique brands in the fitness & wellbeing sector.

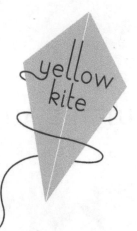

books to help you live a good life

Join the conversation and tell
us how you live a #goodlife

🐦 @yellowkitebooks
📘 YellowKiteBooks
📌 Yellow Kite Books
📷 YellowKiteBooks